Bodies in a Broken World

Studies in Social Medicine

Alan M. Brandt and Larry R. Churchill, *editors*

Bodies in a Broken World

Women Novelists of Color and the Politics of Medicine

Ann Folwell Stanford

The University of North Carolina Press
Chapel Hill and London

Designed by Cameron Poulter
Set in Ellington
by Keystone Typesetting, Inc.

The paper in this book meets the guidelines for permanence and durability
of the Committee on Production Guidelines for Book Longevity of the Council
on Library Resources.

Library of Congress Cataloging-in-Publication Data
Stanford, Ann Folwell.
Bodies in a broken world : women novelists of color and the politics of
medicine / by Ann Folwell Stanford.
p. cm. — (Studies in social medicine)
Includes bibliographical references and index.
ISBN 0-8078-2805-X (alk. paper)—ISBN 8078-5480-8 (pbk. : alk. paper)
1. American fiction—20th century—History and criticism. 2. Medicine in
literature. 3. Women and literature—United States—History—20th century.
4. American fiction—Minority authors—History and criticism. 5. American
fiction—Women authors—History and criticism. 6. Ethnic groups in
literature. 7. Body, Human, in literature. 8. Minorities in literature. 9. Sick
in literature. I. Title. II. Series.
PS374.M433 S73 2003
813'.509356—dc21
2003004081

Portions of this work appeared earlier, in somewhat different form, as " 'Death
is a skipped meal compared to this': Food and Hunger in Toni Morrison's
Beloved," in *Scenes of the Apple: Food and the Female Body in Nineteenth- and
Twentieth-Century Women's Writing*, ed. Patricia Moran and Tamar Heller
(Albany: State University of New York Press, 2003), and "Mechanisms of
Disease: Health, Illness, and the Limits of Medicine in Three African-American
Women's Novels," *NWSA Journal* 6.1 (1994), published by Indiana Univer-
sity Press, and are reprinted here with permission. Acknowledgment of
permission to reprint other previously published material may be found at the
end of the book.

cloth   07 06 05 04 03   5 4 3 2 1
paper   07 06 05 04 03   5 4 3 2 1

For my parents, Chris and Bill Folwell,
for my son, Ben,
and—always—for my partner,
Ora Schub

Contents

Acknowledgments

In 1987 while I was working on a dissertation on Gwendolyn Brooks's poetry, I was offered a fellowship to teach in the Department of Social Medicine at the University of North Carolina at Chapel Hill. It was a lucky and good two years for me, in which many of the ideas in this book began their gestation. I was privileged to work with a gifted, warm faculty and staff who took me in and treated me as one of their own. I am especially grateful to Larry Churchill, Martha Edwards, Sue Estroff, Gail Henderson, Jackie Jones, Nancy King, Don Madison, and Glenn Wilson. Larry Churchill first approached me a few years later about writing this book, and I have appreciated his and Alan Brandt's patience and support, as well as Sian Hunter's at UNC Press. I am also grateful to Trudier Harris for her support and friendship over the years, and for Pat and K. V. Dey, who housed me for nearly a year while I commuted between Chapel Hill and Chicago.

At DePaul I am continually amazed at the richness of the collegial and intellectual community within which I find myself. Marixsa Alicea has consistently challenged and illuminated my thinking throughout this project; this book would have been very different— and diminished—without her. I also appreciate extensive comments on different chapters from Mechtild Hart and Ann Russo. Marixsa, Mechtild, and Ann are fine examples of engaged activist scholars and have taught me a great deal, as have Alicia Alvarez, Anghesom Atsbaha, Deborah Wood Holton, Susan Reed, Derise Tolliver, and Tom Drexler, who are among the many colleagues whose friendship, commitment to social justice, and intellectual gifts remind me regularly how grateful I am to be at DePaul.

Wherever she has been located, Diane Price Herndl has provided encouragement and hours of reading from the inception of this project through its finish—I am more grateful than I can say. I am also grateful to former and current members of the Chicago Narrative and Medicine Group, especially Suzanne Poirier, Barbara Sharf, and Kathryn Montgomery, whose friendship was one of the happy surprises when I moved to Chicago in 1990 and continues to be a source of goodness in my life. Nancy Dew Taylor and Rita Charon provided me with useful comments on a shorter version of chapter 7, which was published in *Literature and Medicine.*

Several years ago Martha Sonnenberg took me on rounds with her at Cook County Hospital, where among other things, I saw AIDS patients from the county jail cuffed and shackled to their beds. It is a vision I won't soon forget. I appreciate Martha's friendship over the years.

Many of the activists in Chicago with whom I am fortunate enough to work—some of whom are academicians as well—provide me with daily proof that the boundaries between the academy and the community are unnecessary: Joanne Archibald, Salome Chasnoff, Mary Ann Corley, Renny Golden, Cheryl Graves, Marvin Lindsey, Erica Meiners, Sr. Patricia Schlosser, Ora Schub, and Zeva Schub, to name only a few. And to the women writers in Cook County Jail who have always reminded me to make a way out of no way, I say thank you.

My former dean at the School for New Learning, David Justice; my current dean, Susanne Dumbleton; and the University Research Council at DePaul provided me with research leaves and overall support, without which I would not have been able to complete this project. I am also very grateful to my research assistant, Carmen White, whose help tracking down errant footnotes at the eleventh hour was a sure sanity-saver. Ron Maner at UNC Press and copyeditor Stephanie Wenzel have been enormously helpful.

And thanks always to Maureen Newton, dear friend for decades. I also owe a debt of gratitude to Theo Pintzuk. My parents, Bill and Chris Folwell, continually inspire me with their sense of adventure, curiosity, and humor. Thanks to David Stanford for years of support and ongoing friendship, to Mark and Kathy Folwell, and to my sister, Susie Folwell, and my daughter-in-law Becky Stanford. My partner Ora Schub's unswerving commitment to social justice has been one of the best reasons I have completed this book. One of the other best reasons has been my son, Ben Stanford, of whom I am prouder than any academic achievement.

Bodies in a Broken World

Introduction

They say behind the mountains are more mountains. Now I know it's true.
I also know there are timeless waters, endless seas, and lots of people in this
world whose names don't matter to anyone but themselves.
—Edwidge Danticat, "Children of the Sea"

Amla which I too would like to take somedays to help bear the pain that
cannot be changed, pain growing slow and huge like a monsoon cloud which
if you let it will blot out the sun.
—Chitra Banerjee Divakaruni, *The Mistress of Spices*

I was recently in Suchitoto, El Salvador, visiting two projects for women's wellness and advocacy. In a rambling, somewhat crumbling building, with rooms arranged around a courtyard filled with lush tropical flowers and ferns in this rainy season, I was invited to the doorway of a room where I heard the strains of quiet, relaxing music and saw a candle flickering. A Salvadoran woman, a *campesina* who had worked in subsistence farming all her life, was lying face down on a table as another Salvadoran gently worked with her patient's body, using acupressure and healing massage techniques. I was inside the walls of Capacitar, a trauma center for women who live in Suchitoto and the surrounding villages. This region, at the foot of Guazapa Volcano, was one of the most heavily conflictive during the brutal course of the twelve-year Salvadoran civil war. These women have seen massacres, endured occupation, and suffered torture. They have lived in anguish over disappeared family members and have seen the country's corrupt government fail time after time to meet the points of the 1992 peace accords (or as some Salvadorans prefer to call it more accurately, "the cessation of armed conflict"). In addition, they have survived earthquakes (one in 1986 and two in 2001, with their devastating sequelae and thousands of aftershocks) and the slow, at times absent, response of a government that has historically cared more about public relations than the health of its people. They are

1

also surviving, in many cases, the brutality of escalating domestic violence. At Capacitar the women know what many of the novelists I have studied for this book know: health is inextricably bound to social conditions. They have taken it upon themselves to learn about the resources they have within their own hands and minds to promote health rather than wait for the (perhaps) monthly visit from a governmental health worker.[1] They know that the physical ailments each of them suffers are almost always rooted in their material and social reality. It is evident all over the world—from Chicago's jails to Palestine's occupied territories to Colombia's militarized *campos*— that the boundaries delineating phenomena such as war, hunger, violence, poverty, literacy, and health are arbitrary and overlapping.

A very real urgency underlies each of the fictive representations considered in this book. The texts do not simply advocate a shift from a biomedical to a biopsychosocial model (no small matter itself) but reconceptualize the nature of illness and health.[2] Angela Davis, discussing African American women's health, insists that "while our health is undeniably assaulted by natural forces frequently beyond our control, all too often the enemies of our physical and emotional well-being are social and political."[3] Placed in a political and social context, illness and health offer a broad, complex, and often messy array of dimensions, and as others have argued, "medicine and society are not separate, independent forces, one determining the other; they are interdependent and shape each other."[4]

This is no news to feminists. Indeed, feminist medical ethics strives to locate the patient in her or his sociocultural context, not simply by way of an addition to the ethical process, but as an epistemological prerequisite to it.[5] Susan Sherwin argues that a feminist framework for medical ethics would understand that "as long as we focus on the merely personal—that is, on an individual encounter with a particular doctor—we cannot see the systematic force of sexist assumptions in our health care institutions."[6] Sherwin insists that a feminist perspective not only would focus on the social and political contexts of individuals but also "will attend to the power relations that structure the relevant interactions."[7] Stating that medical ethics must pay attention to what she calls "housekeeping issues" rather than "crisis issues," Virginia Warren also points to the need for examining more closely "how philosophical moral debates are conducted, especially how ulterior motives influence our beliefs and arguments."[8] Warren says a feminist perspective would bring new questions to medical ethics, and she outlines four categories of interrogation: "(1) inequalities, (2) sexist occupational roles, (3) personal issues, and (4) relationship issues that do not involve deciding the winner of power struggles."[9]

Like Sherwin and Warren, Howard Waitzkin (who does not identify himself as a feminist but shares many feminist perspectives) argues that there is a relationship between the "personal troubles" a patient brings to the medical encounter and the "social issues" in patients' lives, although those connections are not always visible or evident.[10] "On the one hand, medical discourse usually does not attend to institutional causes of suffering. This orientation leads health professionals to overlook social change as a possible therapeutic option. On the other hand, when doctors do consider institutional problems in their encounters with patients, the intervention frequently serves to support the status quo."[11] Appropriate motives notwithstanding, "in trying to help their patients, doctors often find ways that patients can adjust to troubling social conditions."[12] As does Waitzkin, Paul Farmer warns medicine against allowing "social inequalities" to become "embodied as bad health outcomes."[13] Along similar lines, Michael Taussig asserts that "by denying the human relations embodied in symptoms, signs, and therapy, we not only mystify them but we also reproduce a political ideology in the guise of a science of (apparently) 'real things'—biological and physical thinghood."[14] In other words, medical treatment all too often becomes the means of reproducing and/or maintaining systems of oppression.

It is up to medicine, Waitzkin says, to help patients make connections between social issues and personal troubles, and one way that can be done is to contextualize their illnesses more directly. Waitzkin's argument calls for an intentional social intervention on the part of physicians. This kind of intervention, it seems to me, can sustain itself *only* within the structure of a multifaceted community-based model of health care where the institution of medicine is only a part, albeit an important part, of a more far-reaching health care enterprise. In this setting the body's health is inseparable from that body's relationship to the greater community (or world) and its health. While Waitzkin and Taussig examine medical discourse and the doctor-patient encounter, Sherwin looks at the failings in traditional medical ethics and calls for a feminist perspective that sees as one of its goals the empowerment of patients—especially people of color and U.S. women of European descent.[15]

In May 1998 Chicago's Ravenswood Hospital was the focus of controversy and national outrage when fifteen-year-old Christopher Sercye was left to die of gunshot wounds in an alley as emergency room workers refused to treat him, pointing to Ravenswood's policy that strictly forbade personnel from leaving the building to help patients. About thirty minutes later a frustrated police officer finally took out a wheelchair and brought the young man in, but he died from complications due to bleeding from a perforated aorta shortly thereafter. Nationally, Ravenswood stood as a symbol of medicine's institutional paralysis and its remove from human community. Ravenswood was singled out, to be sure: President Bill Clinton threatened to pull $57 million in Medicare and Medicaid funding from Ravenswood if it did not take steps to ensure that "tragedies like the death of . . . Christopher Sercye are never repeated."[16] There were calls for the city to take another look at the overall trauma response system and for Ravenswood to revise its policies, but many observers wondered what had happened to medicine as an institution. A neighbor of Ravenswood Hospital expressed what many in Chicago and the nation were thinking: "If we cannot be responsible as human beings to help each other, it's a shame. . . . Nobody should have to lie in an alley dying next to a hospital."[17]

It is no secret that the institution of medicine is struggling under the heavy hand of managed care and its regulations, privatization of many public systems of care, and decreased government spending for welfare. So, too, are those it was created to serve. It is old news that managed care limits both patients' and physicians' options. It also both benefits from and is hampered by a growing number of (expensive) technological developments. A recent call to action from the Massachusetts-based Ad Hoc Committee to Defend Health Care states in apocalyptic tones its assessment of the current situation:

> Mounting shadows darken our calling and threaten to transform healing from a covenant into a business contract. Canons of commerce are displacing dictates of healing, trampling our professions' most sacred values. Market medicine treats patients as profit centers. The time we are allowed to spend with the sick shrinks under the pressure to increase [throughout], as though we were dealing with industrial commodities rather than afflicted human beings in need of compassion and caring. . . . And patients worry that their physician's judgment and advice are guided by the corporate bottom line. . . . At the same time, the ranks of the uninsured continue to grow.[18]

Thus the economics of medicine complicates even more the already complex class, gender, racial, ethnic, sexual, and other socially constructed difference in the patient-doctor relationship.

While my primary focus in this study is on how women novelists of color in the United States refigure the body in illness and health and, in so doing, critique contemporary medicine and society, another question has animated my readings. As I studied the texts, I began wondering how these writers might also map out contours of possibility for institutional medicine. What good news might be embedded within the critiques? I hope that the stories these writers tell might illuminate social practice—within medicine and within the broader community. For if one thing is clear from my readings of these novels, contemporary medicine cannot work effectively in a vacuum, nor can it be solely responsible for addressing the myriad social and political issues that working with a broad array of patients raises.

Much of what I have written in this book is about bad news, however. These novels contain strong critiques, challenges to oppressive, ignorant, and unjust practices within medicine. But behind some of the criticism is, I believe, a deep concern for the hearts and souls not only of the patients but of the women and men who work with them as health care providers. What might these writers want to say to them? What ways are these writers asking us to rethink, not just the practice of medicine, but the institution and its role, its situatedness within the community?

In her novel *The Mistress of Spices*, Chitra Banerjee Divakaruni creates a woman who heals with spices, a woman who has undergone mystical transformation and is able to work healing magic through her ability to communicate with both her patients and the spices she uses to heal them. Living and working in a small storefront, Tilo's healing powers are contingent on her absolute allegiance to her craft and the spices. She is enjoined by her teachers never to leave the physical boundaries of the shop and never to become involved with her patients' lives beyond it.

Little by little, curiosity, connection with her patients, and loneliness drive Tilo to transgress the boundaries and to walk among the community, where she sees the contexts in which her patients live and meets their families. Eventually she falls in love. Faced with the choice of being an ageless healer (for that is part of her gift; she will always be beautiful as long as she stays within the confines of the spice shop and her calling) or an aging mortal, she chooses life with a newfound lover and is forever cut off from the spices' communion and power. Indeed, her beauty quickly fades, but she has become human. Many questions remain unanswered: Will her work as a healer continue? Will she simply get lost in the mundane and quotidian life of a woman in love? This is not clear at the end of the novel, but Tilo's move out of isolation, motivated by curiosity about the lives of the patients she has cared for throughout the years, is not unlike the many strands of narrative bioethics, biopsychosocial emphases, and medical training that stress patients' stories—representing a shift from the illusion of privileged (and isolated) knowing and into partnership with the community and a wider range of epistemologies rife with potential and challenges.

Medicine has long been a collaborative, though hierarchical, enterprise: chaplains, social workers, nurses, technicians, and physicians all work toward the amelioration of a patient's health. Less energy has been spent on moving beyond clinic or hospital walls. In the face of worsening poverty, rising crime, and the obscene profits of managed care, medicine is in danger of becoming the patient itself. By believing the myth that the only healing, the only way to health is through institutionalized medicine, practitioners run the risk of missing spaces of creative possibility, spaces permitted precisely by the careful listening to stories of the marginalized and oppressed. But those spaces are all too often cast as pathologies, or problems to be solved (that will, for the "solvers," become avenues for burnout or cynicism). Like Gloria Naylor's superrational, technologically proficient character, George, who joins hands too late with the mystical rootworker, Mama Day, and loses his life, medicine is, I believe, in danger of losing its soul and its effectiveness. Instead, with the focus on listening to stories and paying attention to the contexts of patients, it is offered the opportunity to join forces with communities and improbable partners in the healing enterprise by seeing itself as one of a spectrum of healing possibilities.

In the last thirty or so years, scholars, writers, and practitioners have been rethinking the practice of medicine, calling for a balance between detachment and attachment, rather than a strict adherence to a more so-called objective science. Feminists, Marxist scholars, bioethicists, medical anthropologists and sociologists have variously and in different ways called for physicians to pay attention to the life context of the patient, particularly those life contexts that are usually relegated to the offices of social workers, priests, or judges. The more recent surge of work that looks at the connection between narrative and ethics also insists that ethical decision making can never be divorced from the stories of patients and their families.[19]

I am concerned about what it is that doctors and other medical practitioners are supposed to do with the stories they may hear, especially stories that are not familiar or whose narratives do not follow the rough contours of their own. In many cases the contexts of poor, uneducated, uninsured, nonmainstream patients will be harrowing, overwhelming, and likely more complex than those of their more privileged counterparts. What are physicians to do with the knowledge they will gain from listening to stories of oppression, injustice, and hopelessness? Howard Brody raises the issue in thinking about the ongoing work of bioethics:

> At a minimum, bioethics must be working with whoever within medicine is listening to start to think about what will be needed when the supposed sanctuary of invulnerability and "detached concern" ceases to exist. We have, for instance, usually thought of institutional ethics committees as multidisciplinary panels of inquiry or tools for crafting consensus about moral issues. We may have to begin thinking about them much more as potential sources for emotional and social support for caregivers who are truly willing to confront and to be altered by the story of the patient's suffering.[20]

I remember a fourth-year student in a Chicago-area medical school where I was teaching a course on literature and the politics of medicine a few years ago. One day after class he waited until the other students had left the room and asked if he could tell me a story. He had, in his first year, been asked to take a patient off the respirator so that she could die. Once he had extubated the patient, as expected, she died. The student told me that he had never discussed this with anyone because he was so tormented over the possibility that he had committed murder. He had not been able to reconcile his religious convictions and fulfilling his duty as a first-year medical student. Only three years later had he been able to bring up the subject. Where was the community within and outside medicine to help this student come to terms with exigencies of the profession and his own spiritual and emotional life? The fact that he was of South Asian descent or that his religious background was not mainstream may have played a role, but what was overridingly important is that he had not felt safe in discussing what he perceived as a professional weakness, on one hand, and the possibility that he had transgressed an ethical boundary, on the other. Indeed David Hilfiker has written eloquently about the personal cost of medical mistakes that go unacknowledged and unresolved, but what of medical actions that are not mistakes but nevertheless cause guilt and a sense of moral uncertainty? What kind of community—within and beyond medicine—exists in which physicians and other health care providers can humanely function with one another, with their patients, and with themselves?

Another story: Filmmaker John Sayles recounts how his friend, novelist Francisco Goldman, told Sayles about his uncle who was a doctor in Guatemala. He had become involved in an international health program only to find a few years later that most of his students "whom he had sent off in good faith to serve as barefoot doctors in the poorer communities, had been murdered by the very government that claimed to support the program."[21] Inspired by Goldman's story, Sayles made his 1998 film *Men With Guns*, in which a wealthy physician, Humberto Fuentes, lives an isolated and privileged life in an unnamed country that could just as easily be Colombia, Guatemala, or El Salvador as Chiapas. Fuentes has paid little attention to the political and social realities of his country but considers his greatest achievement to have been his participation as a teacher in an international health program, in which he trained young students to work as doctors in poor villages throughout his country. Despite an ailing heart, he is drawn by curiosity, like Divakaruni's Tilo, to venture into the world to see for himself the legacy he has left his country. At each village, he sees poverty and disease and discovers that every one of his students has been killed— some horribly—by "men with guns." As the journey grows more complex and the buffer of privilege that protected Fuentes from such knowledge is stripped away, he becomes more and more ill and finally dies when he reaches the one village where, he has been told, men with guns do not exist. Once Fuentes ventures out of the safety of his privilege and isolation, he cannot sustain the journey without a just and compassionate community to support him. In his world, there are no social structures, no community that holds itself accountable for the suffering of its people. Fuentes's students end up sacrificed, as does Fuentes himself.

What happens when medicine ventures into the world? In these novels that take medicine to task around issues of racism, sexism, classism, and other injustices, where is the good news? My contention is that if medicine is to heed the words of these writers—and I believe it should—to become more engaged in the community, to become more involved in the struggle for social justice, it cannot possibly continue in the same models. It certainly cannot enter the struggle alone. Medicine must open its doors not only to the sick of its communities but also to those who are well, who have other ways of envisioning health and healing. The novels I have read for this study consistently challenge medicine not to operate out of a heroic Lone Ranger model and to begin to open itself to alternative voices and models of healing and etiology. In addition, however, the implication of my readings of these works is that medicine cannot and should not be the fall guy for the world's messes. Nor is it possible for medicine to be the sole cure for them. I read these books for clues as to how medicine and the community might come together to make medicine more of a focused and rooted practice that begins to approach the spirit of the World Health Organization's definition of health. Not only do the novels suggest the need for medicine to become more accountable to the communities it serves, but those communities must also become more accountable to medicine if it is ever to engage in the struggle for social justice. What social structures support caregivers who confront their patients' devastating realities?

Where is the community when a homeless person who has not eaten for days enters the emergency room with a gangrenous foot? Where is the community when nearly 35 percent of women seeking emergency room care are battered? It is too easy to demand that the institution and its caregivers are to move toward a more socially engaged practice without demanding just structures and supports within our communities.

This book is not a how-to manual. The novels I have read do not offer answers to the many issues they illuminate, but within them are, I believe, tracings of possibilities for medicine and society to rethink illness and health and their relationship to the community, as well as the connection between social justice and health. I have chosen to focus on only a few novels that provide a wide array of views into medicine and health—novels by African American, Latina, and Native American women. Noticeably missing are novels by women of Arab, Asian, and Pacific Rim descent. This is due only to the narrow scope of my project. The field is rich for exploration. I have chosen novels written by U.S. writers because I wanted to focus on domestic health issues primarily, but the potential for a similar study of women writers around the world is great. I would love to see more work done on Nawal el Saadawi, Keri Hulme, Angelés Mastrata, and Buchi Emecheta, for example, and hope that this book will be a catalyst for further research in these areas.[22] I have obviously also not written about every U.S. woman writer of color who deals with medicine. An entire chapter or chapters could be devoted to Gayl Jones or to Alice Walker, for example.[23] I am struck by Dorothy Roberts's argument that "because women of color experience the intersection of gender and racial oppression, they may have unique critical insights to offer" the study of medicine. She goes on to say that "the perspective of poor women of color . . . can uncover the way in which the practice of medicine . . . perpetuates hierarchies of power [and] can highlight women's forms of resistance to medical control, and can propose a vision for transforming medical ethics and the health care system."[24] While the novelists in this study are not necessarily "poor" women of color, and although novels or novelists cannot "speak for" poor women of color, I believe that the textual constructions illuminate many of the critical insights Roberts mentions, and that these insights are precisely those without which no real transformation in medicine will ever occur.

The book is loosely divided into two sections. The bulk of each chapter contains literary analysis but concludes with a brief coda that addresses the relevance of the work to medicine directly. The first five chapters deal with individual characters and their illnesses and/or journeys toward healing. In Chapter 1, Toni Cade Bambara's *The Salt Eaters*, Paule Marshall's *Praisesong for the Widow*, and Gloria Naylor's *The Women of Brewster Place* all have characters that become ill because they have lost touch with important aspects of their history and communities. Always, however, there are political and social factors at work: the interlocking categories of sexism, racism, classism, and other injustices. Their illnesses are figured in different ways—physically, mentally, and spiritually—but the authors frequently blur the boundaries. Healing for the characters includes remembering and reconnecting with their histories, as it also does for Tayo, the main character in Leslie Marmon Silko's *Ceremony*, the subject of Chapter 2. Battle-fatigued and near nervous collapse, Tayo learns to resist the dominant narrative of his illness and to understand its roots in social injustice, finding healing through traditional indigenous means.

Continuing to make and to intensify the connection between sick bodies and unjust, sick worlds, Toni Morrison complicates memory, as it becomes oppressive and injurious to the slave body in *Beloved*. Chapter 3 looks at how Sethe struggles against the memory of slavery and of her baby's murder at her own hands, and how she is almost lost as that baby comes back to haunt her in the form of an embodied ghost—her murdered child—who represents racism's annihilating function. While there are no doctors in *Beloved*, and the illnesses represented seem more psychological than physical, Sethe's near-starvation and the returned ghost-child's obsessive eating inspire useful contemplation about how history becomes written as

illness and dysfunction on oppressed bodies. Racism is also an annihilating factor in Native and African American female characters'
bodies in Louise Erdrich's novel *Tracks* and Morrison's *The Bluest
Eye*, and the discussion in Chapter 4 focuses on the consequences of
failing to resist dominant, racist narratives and the ways medicine
wittingly or unwittingly maintains those narratives. Chapter 5 looks
at novels in which characters break through the silence and trauma of
domestic and sexual violence and create new language and narratives. Sandra Cisneros's "Woman Hollering Creek," Bebe Moore
Campbell's *Your Blues Ain't Like Mine*, and Sapphire's *Push* insist, as
do all the novels in this section of the book, that the characters have
within themselves the tools for much of their own healing, but that
healing happens within the context of what Robert Bellah calls a
"community of memory."[25] Such a community "is involved in retelling its story, its constitutive narrative," but such a community "will
also tell painful stories of shared suffering that sometimes creates
deeper identities than success."[26] Moreover, all of the illnesses and
injuries the characters suffer are rooted in historical atrocity and
social injustice.

The focus of the second section shifts to novels that hold medicine
itself under the microscope. Chapter 6 takes up the subject of narrative ethics and uncertainty through a reading of Ana Castillo's *So Far
from God* and Gloria Naylor's *Mama Day*. Both novels (especially
Castillo's) continue to make the connection between social structures
of oppression and illness, but they also raise important questions for
medicine about epistemology—and healing. Medicine becomes the
patient in Leslie Marmon Silko's *Almanac of the Dead*, as practitioners
are implicated in an increasingly profitable traffic in human organs
and as civil wars in Mexico make human cadavers readily available.
Silko raises the question of what constitutes human worth in this
troubling novel, the subject of Chapter 7. If the society Silko creates
in *Almanac* is troubling, the one Octavia Butler constructs in *Parable
of the Sower* and *Parable of the Talents*, the subject of chapter 8, is
positively nightmarish. In these novels Butler creates the horrible
world of "the Pox," in which disease and human cruelty rule. A small

band of refugees, one of whom is a physician, come together to create a community, and thus the seeds of possibility are born. In *Talents* the community members are taken captive, and many are murdered. After the survivors escape, they eventually reconfigure as a powerful force, having survived the Pox, and begin to set up new frontiers, dreaming of new possibilities not only on Earth but among the stars as well.

And so we are left with possibility. None of the novels I have chosen to write about provides easy—or any—answers, something that readers may find frustrating. What they will do is challenge readers, medical and nonmedical alike, to think about illness and healing as something we are all responsible for. If health is contingent on social good, on factors such as education, food, shelter, and safety, institutional medicine cannot "provide" or "deliver" it (despite the splashy advertising of hospitals, managed care companies, and the like). Health is rooted in the world's body, as the voices in the novels attest. These voices are strong, at times enraged, and resist or demonstrate the fiercely dehumanizing aspects of medicine. But they also embed their stories in dehumanizing worlds. What I hope readers will hold in mind is that it is not only patients who bear the scars of such dehumanization (although they may bear them most intensely) but ultimately caregivers and practitioners of medicine and the communities within which they practice as well.

Wasted Blood and Rage

Social Pathologies and the Limits of Medicine in Toni Cade
Bambara's *The Salt Eaters*, Paule Marshall's *Praisesong for the Widow*,
and Gloria Naylor's *The Women of Brewster Place*

1

> Are you sure, sweetheart, that you want to be well?
> —Toni Cade Bambara, *The Salt Eaters*

> The problem is
> to connect, without hysteria, the pain
> of any one's body with the pain of the body's world.
> —Adrienne Rich, "Contradictions: Tracking Poems, 18"

During the 1970s and 1980s, fiction by African American women writers intensified a focus on the connections between politics and illness. Toni Cade Bambara's *The Salt Eaters* (1981), Paule Marshall's *Praisesong for the Widow* (1983), and Gloria Naylor's *The Women of Brewster Place* (1983) challenge medicine into rethinking its role in healing.[1] All of these texts probe the complexities of private, individual illness but refuse to separate illness from its social context, brushing against the grain of strict biomedical accounts.[2] In these novels the medical profession is frequently absent or relegated to the margins of the text. Constructing "thick descriptions" of illness, each of these writers levels her gaze at the problematics, indeed the possibility, of individual healing in a world—a global community—that itself bears symptoms of terminal illness.

Shifting the site of onset from the body to the world—the social and cultural community within which individuals live—these texts foreground the connections between an individual's physical body and her private as well as collective history. In these stories, living human bodies pay the price for and carry within them the symptoms of a sick world. The disorders causing the symptoms are vague, unnamed, and thus resist biomedical classification and control. Velma

Henry, the main character in *The Salt Eaters*, has just attempted suicide; Avey Johnson, in *Praisesong for the Widow*, has vague gastrointestinal symptoms (also imitating cardiac distress); and Ciel Turner, in *The Women of Brewster Place*, is feverish and dying.

Existing in almost mimetic relation to the world's violence, the body becomes the site of profound struggle that much African American women's fiction inscribes as illness. In thus positing a reciprocity between world illness and body illness, the texts do not discount medical models but redirect them, insisting that health in a world caught in its own complicated webs of oppression and hegemony is an impossible dream, at best available only to a select few. The fiction of Bambara, Marshall, and Naylor, while engaging in an indirect critique of medicine, also lays bare the relationships between Howard Waitzkin's notion of personal troubles and social issues that exist in many medical encounters and ethical deliberations, thus linking the two. In addition, the novels construct a vision of health rooted in social justice, a vision that thematizes the concerns of feminist medical ethics. This vision is rooted not only in social justice, however, but in a commitment to personal and community empowerment as well.

Just what that empowerment might mean is precisely what *The Salt Eaters*, *Praisesong for the Widow*, and *The Women of Brewster Place* explore. Each novel constructs a character who experiences debilitating symptoms from which she must recover before reentering a world that itself remains sick. The novels insist that understanding the connection between sick bodies and a sick world is crucial to making a workable vision equipped for urgent social change and global healing. Individual healing, far from providing a privatistic cure, enables its subjects to move beyond a narrow understanding of individual illness to become potential world healers themselves. Refusing to *name* the illness, these novels render the concept of disease problematic and resist the definitions that would serve as access points for institutionalized, technological medicine, insisting that in some cases, medicine's tools are simply inappropriate or that the cure may actually be worse than the illness. Although access to medical care is a vital concern for women of color and, indeed, many marginalized and uninsured or underinsured people in the United States,[3] in these texts the terms of hegemony are reversed as medicine is closed out of the diagnostic and healing process. Without biomedical labels, these illnesses are out of medicine's reach and remain in the domain of people and communities best equipped to understand them, those who have the wisdom and skill to facilitate a healing that is not and cannot be separate from social context. Resisting traditional medicine, these texts avoid categories or labels that function as mechanisms of power and strategies of control.[4]

As *The Salt Eaters* begins, Velma Henry sits bleary-eyed and ragged on a stool in the Southwest Community Infirmary with Minnie Ransom, "the fabled healer of Claybourne, Georgia," surrounded by twelve spiritual adepts, various clinic patients, and a bored, somewhat nervous group of visiting interns, nurses, and technicians. Literally on the periphery of the circle, they (along with the director and one of the attending physicians at the infirmary) are referred to only occasionally as the novel progresses. At the beginning of the session, one of the doctors defiantly mumbles to himself, but loud enough for the others to hear, "I swear by Apollo the physician . . . by Aesculapius, Hygeia and Panacea . . . and I take to witness all the gods, all the goddesses . . . to keep according to my ability and my judgment the following [Hippocratic] oath" (*Salt*, 55). Eleanor Traylor notes that "the brilliant Dr. Meadows who has masterminded Velma's therapeutic surgery . . . regards the healing ritual of the Master's Mind with contempt, skeptical of all experience unverified by the code of a closed system which has become his logic."[5] Now that Velma's self-inflicted wounds have been bandaged, a different kind of healing must take place, but it is a healing with which the medical establishment, represented by Dr. Meadows and the other physicians, is clearly uncomfortable. For among other things, the novel resists any attempt to separate mind, spirit, body, and social context. Unlike the treatments described in many of the other novels examined in this study, Minnie Ransom's healing sessions take place *within* the clinic walls and with medical people present. A partnership (however uneasy) as well as an accountability exists. Although Dr. Meadows thinks that Velma is a psychiatric case, she is not referred away but handed over to Minnie Ransom, who administers another kind of treatment, asking from the outset if Velma really wants "the weight" of being well. Minnie exemplifies the attitude toward healing that feminist ethics calls for, an interest in fostering agency, an attitude that questions "how to strengthen the patient's agency, how to help her to make medical decisions that will serve her well."[6] Implicit in Minnie Ransom's question is the insistence that Velma be willing to take responsibility for healing and its implications— being well.

It is not just that Velma is tired out, "stressed," but that the context of her stress—that which drove her to slashed wrists and the "carbon cave" of her gas stove—represents a complex network of sociopolitical as well as emotional factors. And the context *is* complicated. The imagery of splitting, splinters, and disjunction characterizes not only Velma's experience but the nature of the illness attributed to the community and the broader world as well. Velma is consumed with long-standing anger, fear, and increasing alienation from her cultural and historical past, even as she works to maintain and move herself and her already progressive community beyond a narrow understanding of social justice. Underlying and permeating Velma's and her community's collective exhaustion is an oppressive social system and world order within which health is at best dubious.

The Salt Eaters rests on the assumption that the world is sick and that in order to survive, human beings must be about the business of healing it through social, political, cultural, and spiritual channels. There is an ecology at stake, however. On one hand, when individuals ignore their own health—be that spiritual, physical, or emotional— they cannot fully engage in building a healthier world. On the other hand, the notion of an individual health divorced from community is an illusion. In most of the texts examined in this study, those characters who heal experience that healing within community and are restored to their communities when well, even when those communities themselves will need work—world healing. Sarah Hoagland's

notion of "autokoenony" is useful here. Hoagland says she constructed the word to mean "the self in community" that "involved
each of us making choices . . . each of us having a self-conscious sense
of ourselves as moral agents in a community of other self-conscious
moral agents."[7] The model consists of individuals as components of a
community, or more likely, communities, functioning together, in
different ways at different times, as a human ecosystem.

Velma, a veritable superwoman, remains captive to expectations
that she be individually responsible for upholding the collective
good. This is not to say she works in a vacuum; she has many friends
and belongs to collectives and political organizations, but her sense
of connection to her past, to those persons with whom she lives and
those causes she seeks to serve, is weakened by her excessive reliance
on herself. Velma embodies the American ethic of individualism in
which, as Robert Bellah says, "the self has become the main form
of reality."[8] She is disconnected from her past and desperately attempts to hold her life together through unaided self-will. In the
meantime, her life totters on the brink of disaster. What is puzzling
about Velma is that, on the surface, she *looks* connected to the community. She has, with her husband, Obie, founded and directed the
now-fragmented and troubled Academy of Seven Arts. In addition,
she actively participates in a women's political caucus and a women's
arts collective, as well as in her own marriage and child rearing; all
this is compounded by the stress of a full-time job as a computer
programmer at a company where she is regularly interrogated for
security leaks. Plagued by anger, exhausted, and chronically un-
prepared for her menstrual bleeding ("wasted blood and rage" [*Salt*,
34]), Velma wants to climb inside an empty jar where there is only
light, where she can be "sealed and unavailable to sounds, voices,
cries" (*Salt*, 19).

Velma's attempted suicide is the culmination of an increasing
physical and emotional exhaustion as well as alienation from her
body and her legacy as an African American woman. Not only is she
exhausted from her political endeavors, but Velma runs from frightening visions, "the calling, the caves, the mud mothers, and the

others" (*Salt*, 19) who haunt her prior to her suicide attempt. There is no escape: while worrying about the problems of her community one morning, Velma sees the mud mothers "almost come tumbling out of the mirror naked and tattooed with serrated teeth and hair alive, birds and insects peeping out at her from the mud-heavy hanks of the ancient mothers' hair. And she [flees] feverish and agitated from the room" (*Salt*, 259).

However, as she embarks on a journey of memory and recollection, Velma discovers that those mud mothers—rooted in African culture—call her to a deeper understanding of who she is within the social and historical community from which she comes. Despite her desire to be fully engaged in political struggle, she becomes alienated from herself—from her femaleness and her lineage as an African American. The gap is vast and is mirrored by the community's insensitivity to repressive sexual politics. "Velma [is one who] has worked hard not to hollow out a safe corner . . . of home, family, marriage, and then be less responsive, less engaged" (*Salt*, 241). Ironically, those things that seem healthy in and of themselves—politically engaged worldviews and concomitant action, rootedness in the "movement"— actually contribute to an overall sickness, and the political and institutional splintering Velma has tried to prevent occurs within her:

> [She] thought she knew how to build immunity to the
> sting of the serpent. . . . Thought she knew how to build re-
> sistance, make the journey to the center of the circle, stay
> poised and centered in the work and not fly off, stay cen-
> tered in the best of her people's traditions and not be avail-
> able to madness. . . . Thought the workers of the sixties had
> pulled the Family safely out of the range of the serpent's
> fangs so the workers of the seventies could drain the poi-
> sons, repair damaged tissues, retrain the heartworks, real-
> ign the spine. Thought the vaccine offered by all the
> theorists and activists and clear thinkers . . . would
> take. But amnesia had set in. . . . Something crucial had

been missing from the political/economic/social/
cultural/aesthetic/military/psychosocial/psychosexual
mix. [*Salt*, 258–59]

The terms of physical disease—poisons, damaged tissues, and ineffi-
cient vaccines—thus become figures for social sickness. While Velma
appears to be a suicidal, burned-out community activist who, among
other things, has recently bitten through a drinking glass, the subtext
of that presentation involves the sick community and, indeed, the
globe itself—the sick world from which Velma has "caught" (to rely
on germ theory) her illness.[9] Those social factors from which Velma
has become ill are, the novel argues, deeply embedded in a racist
and sexist society. In effect, the community is both the illness and
the cure. It is from the national community that Velma and countless others experience the effects of racism, sexism, ethnocentrism,
homophobia, classism, and environmental poisoning, and yet one
part of the "cure" lies in a return to a community in which Velma's
relationship to herself is taken as seriously as her relationships with
the world and its inhabitants.

Another important angle of seeing in all three novels discussed
in this chapter draws on African and Afro-Caribbean healing traditions that similarly stress the relational aspects of the human condition: "The understanding of personhood operative within . . . Afro-
Caribbean healing traditions is a fundamentally relational one. The
individual person is defined by a web of relationships that include
not only the extended family, but also the ancestors and the spirits or
saints. . . . The distinction between physical and social maladies is
finally an insignificant one."[10] Part of Velma's healing will involve an
inner journey of "soul gathering" that will help her come to terms
with herself and repair damaged human and social ties, but it will
also prepare her for the difficult world-healing work ahead. To insist
on individual healing first is not to say that the novel advocates a
narcissistic and solipsistic approach to social problems. Far from it.
As Velma comes to the end of the transformative inner journey of
healing, she experiences visions of horrifying futures replete with

nuclear war, melting polar ice caps, and unthinkable violence due to extraordinary deprivation and poverty. In addition, she fuses with an explicitly female and African historical past, experiencing herself "pressed between the sacred rocks, lying on her back under the initiation knife at an age when the female element is circumcised from the boys and the male excised from the girls" (*Salt*, 275–76), and she emerges stronger, more solidly identified with her sexual and cultural heritage. Karla Holloway looks at Velma's healing as a "mediation between history and memory" where Velma becomes reconnected to a network of women, "a community that is simultaneously present and past, temporal and detemporalized."[11] In the eyes of her godmother, Velma finally has now become "ready for training" (*Salt*, 293).

"Soul gathering" will likewise be the means of restoration for Avey Johnson of Paule Marshall's *Praisesong for the Widow*. However, Avey has lost her soul, not to political engagement, but to the socially correct, whitewashed world of immaculate dining rooms, beige crepe de chine, pearls, gloves, and Caribbean cruises.

Omitting mention of doctors and institutional medicine altogether, *Praisesong* chronicles Avey's experience of what appears to be a cardiac or gastrointestinal irregularity but might also be simply dismissed as a psychosomatic complaint. In probing Avey's illness and subsequent healing, the novel refuses to separate the community from individual bodies—or the psychosomatic from the somatic—and in so doing foregrounds the social context of Avey's physical troubles. Avey's real problem, as the novel has it, is the profound emptiness of materialism and social betterment bought at the expense of what Abena P. A. Busia calls "a private history of material acquisition and cultural dispossession."[12] But paradoxically, Avey's emptiness is figured as surfeit; her first symptoms are the uncomfortable sensations of fullness where "her heart was beating thickly . . . [and] her stomach, her entire midsection felt odd" (*Praisesong*, 50); she is subject to a "mysterious clogged and swollen feeling which differed in intensity and came and went at will" (*Praisesong*, 52). She is, as Trudier Harris says, "waterlogged with the pressure of unfulfillment."[13]

From her upper-class suburban home in White Plains to the luxurious cruise liner the *Bianca Pride*, Avey is immersed in white values and culture, having undergone a gradual wearing away of her identity and traditions as a black woman. Indeed, it was the marathon struggle for a white-defined success within the crucible of racism and the immensely difficult climb out of poverty that bled her husband and their marriage of its life. Avey remembers the "small rituals," the "ethos they held in common [that] had reached back beyond her life and beyond Jay's to join them to the vast unknown lineage that had made their being possible" (*Praisesong*, 137), all of which they had lost to the god of the American dream.

Widowed less than a year, Avey has taken no less than six immaculately packed suitcases on a two-week cruise "with a bunch of white folks" (says her indignant daughter [*Praisesong*, 13]) and two of her black coworkers from the State Department of Transportation. On board the *Bianca Pride*, Avey begins to experience unsettling symptoms and has a recurring, disturbing dream in which her Afrocentric Great-aunt Cuney beckons her toward the Ibo Landing in Tatem, the town of her youth ("Come / Won't you come . . . ?" [*Praisesong*, 42]).[14] In the dream, Avey and Aunt Cuney enter a pitched battle over Avey's resistance, and to Avey's horror, the entire neighborhood of North White Plains witnesses the battle.

The disorienting dream and her escalating physical symptoms ultimately prompt Avey to escape the ship, and she disembarks alone in Grenada, where she finally taps the wellspring of grief and anger long blocked within herself. In this section, "Sleepers Wake," Avey comes to mourn not only the death of her husband but the utter waste in his drive for material success, as well as the consequential loss of their joy in each other and their sense of who they were as African Americans. The loss for Avey is simply "Too much! Too much!" (*Praisesong*, 145). Awakening from a long night of rage and grief, Avey takes a walk, becomes dehydrated and exhausted, and meets an old man, Lebert Joseph, in the section "Lave Tete" [Wash your face]. Surprising herself after long conversation, Avey agrees to accompany him on the "Carriacou Excursion," an annual island festival honoring the longtime ancestors—a festival of repentance and community reconciliation. Gay Wilentz, noting the significance of Lebert Joseph's resemblance to the Voodoo loa Papa Legba, describes him as "a spiritual guide who leads Avey back to her heritage . . . who opens the gates to the world of the ancestors for Avey so that she can articulate and move toward reconciliation of the conflicting aspects of her African American personality."[15] Avey's physical distress intensifies as something that "felt like a huge tumor had suddenly ballooned up at her center" (*Praisesong*, 52), and she is cared for by local island women on the boat during the rough crossing. On the way to the remote Carriacou, Avey vomits "in long loud agonizing gushes" (*Praisesong*, 204), the dry retching and "massive contractions doubling her over between the women on the bench" (*Praisesong*, 207).[16]

> The paroxysms repeated themselves with almost no time
> in between for her to breathe. Hanging limp and barely
> conscious over the side of the boat after each one, she
> would try clearing her head, try catching her breath. . . .
> And then she would be hawking, crying, collapsing as her
> stomach convulsed and the half-digested food came gush-
> ing from her with such violence she might have fallen over-
> board were it not for the old women. [*Praisesong*, 205]

Not only is she subject to vomiting and dry retching, but Avey's contractions move "down into the well of her body" (*Praisesong*, 207) and into her bowels, causing uncontrollable diarrhea and unspeakable shame, rendering her briefly unconscious. For Avey, the ride on the *Emmanuel C* to Carriacou becomes a reverse middle passage. As she regains a dim consciousness, she imagines "other [slave] bodies lying crowded in with her in the hot, airless dark. . . . Their moans, rising and falling with each rise and plunge of the schooner, enlarged upon the one filling her head. Their suffering . . . made hers of no consequence" (*Praisesong*, 209).[17] The text appropriates and complicates the terms of biomedicine as Avey's "personal ills" are firmly fixed in a broad social history and the current social ills deriving, in part, from that history. Avey's body bears the marks of an illness that easily traces back to the historical roots of slavery and the current social sickness of poverty, racism, and the seduction of white materialism.[18]

Humiliation is transformed into a liberating humility as Avey, on Carriacou at last, is bathed and oiled by Lebert Joseph's daughter, Rosalie Parvay. Rosalie concludes the ritual with a massage whereby "the warmth, the stinging sensation that was both pleasure and pain . . . reached [Avey's] heart. And as they encircled her heart and it responded, there was the sense of a chord being struck" (*Praisesong*, 224).[19] Strong enough and ready both spiritually and physically, Avey attends the "Big Drum," where she witnesses the "Beg Pardon" and nation dances. This final section brings the novel full circle as Avey experiences the beginning of reconciliation with her past, her heritage, and herself.

Prior to her journey across the water, Avey had remembered an annual picnic in her childhood where, waiting on the dock for the boat, she had experienced "hundreds of slender threads streaming out from her navel and from the place where her heart was to enter those around her. And the threads went out not only to people she recognized from the neighborhood but to those she didn't know as well. . . . She became part of, indeed the center of, a huge wide confraternity" (*Praisesong*, 190, 191).[20] Later, at the Big Drum, Avey reexperiences her childhood vision as "she felt the threads streaming out from the old people around her in Lebert Joseph's yard" (*Praisesong*, 249). She begins to dance, and out of that dancing she learns to "call her nation," to remember, to reconstruct what is good and rich about her past as well as that which has caused suffering. In the act of dancing, she pulls together the strands of resistance that caused her to flee the cruise, the grief over her marriage and alienation from her past, and the reconciliation with the shared stories she has encountered on Carriacou.

For Avey, the myth of Ibo Landing, previously "just" a story, becomes a "narrative of resistance"[21] to white definitions of self and success that have left her life bare and meaningless. The novel suggests that Avey will return home and restore the old homeplace on Tatem Island, revivifying the vital, healing stories and family traditions for herself, her family, and others, and in so doing, she will become a world healer as well. But further, the novel, by constructing symptoms that could be relevant to medicine (it is not hard to imagine someone with Avey's symptoms showing up in an emergency room or making an appointment with her physician), challenges medicine to see beyond narrow biomedical categories. Avey's story suggests the inescapably complex underpinning of what may at first appear to be straightforward physical symptoms.

In Gloria Naylor's *The Women of Brewster Place*, Ciel Turner becomes the survivor of a social and ideological system within which she is almost crushed. Ciel comes to live on Brewster Place, a dead-end street walled off from the rest of the city, "the bastard child of several clandestine meetings between the alderman of the sixth district and the managing director of the Unico Realty Company" (*Brewster Place*, 1). In the same way that Naylor "demonstrate[s] how individual personality is not the determining factor that brings [the women] to this street,"[22] the story demonstrates that individual biological pathology is not the determining factor in all illnesses. For Ciel, the threads of poverty, racism, and sexism weave together to create and mark the fabric of her illness, in which she comes perilously close to death.

Ciel's relief at her husband's return after an eleven-month absence is cut short when she becomes pregnant, Eugene loses his job, and his restless anger resurfaces ("And what the hell we gonna feed it when it gets here, huh—air?" [*Brewster Place*, 95]). "It was all there: the frustration of being left alone, sick, with a month-old baby; her humiliation reflected in the caseworker's blue eyes for the unanswerable 'you can find him to have it, but can't find him to take care of it' smile; the raw urges that crept, uninvited, between her thighs on countless nights; the eternal whys all meshed with the explainable hate and unexplainable love" (*Brewster Place*, 91). This constellation of need drives Ciel to have an abortion as a last-ditch attempt to keep Eugene from leaving her. As she lies on the table, Ciel is impervious to the physician's glib reassurance, "Nothing to it, Mrs. Turner": "It was important that she keep herself completely isolated from these surroundings. All the activities of the past week of her life were balled up and jammed on the right side of her brain, as if belonging to some other woman." It is not surprising that Ciel has trouble "connect[ing] herself up again with her own world" (*Brewster Place*, 95) after the procedure is completed. The abortion becomes a psychic fracture that radically alters Ciel's experience of reality: "Everything seemed to have taken on new textures and colors. . . . The plates felt peculiar in her hands. . . . There was a disturbing split second between someone talking to her and the words penetrating sufficiently to elicit a response" (*Brewster Place*, 95–96). These skewed perceptions recall Velma's visions of the mud mothers and her rage, fear, and consequent desire to seal herself off inside a glass jar. They are also not unlike Avey's shipboard hallucinations, dreams, and troubling physical sensations on board the *Bianca Pride*.

For Ciel, Eugene's announcement that he is leaving compounds the loss occasioned by the abortion. His words cause "a tight, icy knot" to form in her stomach as she turns from the child, Serena, and follows Eugene into the bedroom, begging, demanding that he not leave her. To his abrupt "Why?" Ciel realizes "that to answer that would require that she uncurl that week of her life, pushed safely up into her head, when she had done all those terrible things for that other woman who had wanted an abortion. She and she alone would have to take responsibility for them now." As she begins to see clearly the implications of her life with Eugene, the "poison of reality" begins "to spread through [Ciel's] body like gangrene" (*Brewster Place*, 100) at the same time that she hears her toddler ("the only thing [she had] ever loved without pain" [*Brewster Place*, 93]) scream— electrocuted—in the other room where she had stuck a fork into an outlet in pursuit of a cockroach. Embedded within the narrative of the disintegrating marriage (Eugene's joblessness, Ciel's abortion, their poverty), Serena's death becomes more than an accident or even the result of neglect. The story insists that readers consider the social context of Serena's death: the suffocating web of poverty, racism, and sexism that has shaped Ciel's and Eugene's lives simply cannot be separated from the child's electrocution.

After the double devastation of the unwanted abortion and Serena's death, Ciel refuses to eat, drink, or speak. She becomes even more impenetrable; neither the "sagging chords" from the church organ nor the "droning voice of the black-robed old man behind the coffin" (*Brewster Place*, 101) at the funeral can reach her. Pain has become Ciel's entire world. Elaine Scarry, describing the pain of torture as that which annihilates the world of the sufferer where "world, self, and voice are lost, or nearly lost,"[23] pinpoints the kind of intensity that engulfs Ciel. Her life, indeed her "whole universe," exists "in the seven feet of space between herself and her child's narrow coffin" (*Brewster Place*, 101). And like the coffin, Ciel's pain has become an enclosure: narrow, rigid, and totalizing. Well-meaning guests come to comfort her, but their "impotent words [fly] against the steel edge of her pain, [bleed] slowly, and [return] to die in the senders' throats" (*Brewster Place*, 102).[24]

It is Ciel's friend and neighbor Mattie Michael who sees that Ciel is dying and intervenes. She rushes into the room "like a black Brahman cow, desperate to protect her young" and rocks Ciel in her arms, carrying her back in time and memory, through violent histories shared by ages of women linked to Ciel through mutual suffering: "the fresh blood of sacrificed babies torn from their mother's arms and given to Neptune . . . [to] Dachau, where soul-gutted Jewish mothers swept their children's entrails off laboratory floors . . . [to] the spilled brains of Senegalese infants whose mothers had dashed them on the wooden sides of slave ships. And she rocked on." Mattie rocks Ciel from the larger unframed history of women's brutalization and oppression into the specific frame of her own life, "into her childhood [to] let her see murdered dreams. And she rocked her back, back into the womb, to the nadir of her hurt" (*Brewster Place*, 103). Like Velma and Avey, Ciel must confront her own losses and ghosts. As the "splinter" of pain gives way—"its roots were deep, gigantic, ragged, and they tore up flesh with bits of fat and muscle tissue clinging to them"— Ciel vomits with a violence similar to Avey's

(*Brewster Place*, 103–4). As Rosalie Parvay does for Avey, Mattie bathes Ciel slowly, towels her dry, and lets her cry her rage and grief.[25]

Much as *The Salt Eaters* and *Praisesong* connect illness with a fractured and fracturing community and to the dissociation with individual and collective history, *Brewster Place* links Ciel's illness to the historical pain of countless other women subject to brutal systems.[26] Illness and healing have, in these instances, everything to do with history and social context. Naylor's story, like Bambara's and Marshall's, asks us to consider just what health is, and how—or if—it can exist in a world whose history is written with the blood of oppressed people.

What is medicine's role in healings that seem to be more about social (or psychological) problems than physical ills? Are these stories relevant to medicine? It is commonly acknowledged that as few as 20 percent of the patients seen by physicians have purely medical problems. What of the other 80 percent? What happens when the emergency room doctor encounters her third "Ciel" or "Velma" of the day? What might she see? What might she think? What would her assumptions be? How would those assumptions guide her care of this patient? The novels I have discussed here provide alternative accounts of illnesses that, were they brought to emergency rooms or doctor's offices, would necessarily be translated into biomedical categories. In these fictive accounts, illnesses are spiritual and physical, as well as being rooted in a social context that is itself frequently vast, complex, and intractable. Clearly, medicine cannot escape from the consequences of social injustice and oppression, nor would I argue that it necessarily wants to. The question is whether medicine, in daily encounters with emergency room or clinic patients as well as in dealings with long-term patients, reproduces injustice and oppression or works toward eliminating them.

Although these and the other novels discussed in the first part of this book challenge medicine to look at the context in which patients live and from which their illness may spring—in this chapter, specifically the context of marginalized, oppressed women—they raise the question of medicine's limits and of its place in the healing enterprise. Of the novels discussed above, only one includes the medical establishment in any substantive way, and in this case, the doctors and medical students are clearly on the periphery. Velma's slashed wrists are tended by a physician, but the business of long-term healing is left to Minnie Ransom and the praying community that surrounds her and Velma. These novels begin by decentering medicine, placing it and all of its specialties and technologies in a broader context of healers and factors that affect health, but ultimately they redefine it. In the hands of these authors, medicine becomes a rich complex of approaches, healers, and beliefs. Institutionalized medicine as we know it is not the most important part of such a redefinition.

While Waitzkin argues that "in the long range, contextual change involves nothing short of revolutionary restructuring of social institutions that now create suffering and unhappiness,"[27] he also calls for short-term strategies to change the prevailing medical discourse that tends to marginalize contextual issues. These strategies have to do with interpersonal communication, the kind of inquiry and listening that helps patients make the connection between their personal troubles and social troubles. However, physicians who seriously inquire into the context and social nature of a patient's illness run the risk of being confronted with devastating realities. Surely referral is an important model in helping the physician help her or his patient.

A more important question, however, is how medicine might both use and go beyond the paradigm of referral and toward a more intentional model whereby medicine works in community and sees itself as part of a broader network for social change and the common good. To do this, medicine would have to expand its notion of itself while at the same time encountering its limits. Just as in the novels discussed here each character suffers from a particular kind of disconnection from her community, so, too, does medicine need to deepen its ties to the community, particularly to marginalized communities—to their resources as well as their challenges. Susan Sherwin's feminist ethics would impel medicine to "expand its conceptions of health and health expertise . . . recogniz[ing] social as well as physiological dimensions of health [and] . . . reflect[ing] an understanding of both the moral and health costs of oppression."[28] Dorothy Roberts expands on Sherwin's notions, however, examining the perspective of poor women of color within the doctor-patient relationship and calling for medical ethics to adopt a perspective that is specifically committed to ending disempowerment of women and other oppressed people.[29] For medicine to fulfill this call, it must move further into the community as one agent of social change among many such agents, and so take on a broader role in healing. But at the same time, in entering partnership with the community, medicine would also adopt a realistic view of its limits. It is not and cannot be the cure for all ills.

Does acknowledging limits mean a return to a strict biomedical paradigm that treats only diseased or damaged bodies? Does acknowledging and probing the social context of illness mean doctors must become social workers and agents of change as well? The novels discussed here and the perspectives of feminist medical ethics are troubling and have disturbing implications for medicine. But what they continue to insist, whether or not the individual illness is brought to medicine, is that healing is a multitextured, multilayered dynamic and that medicine's involvement is only a part of that dynamic. For medicine to contribute its part best, it needs to understand and acknowledge its place as one part of a network of factors and forces that contribute to healing. The world is ill. The question these novels raise is how we as a human community will work together to bring it to health.

All We Have to Fight Off Illness and Death

Leslie Marmon Silko's Vision of the Restor(y)ed Community
in *Ceremony*

2

> Where are we moored?
> What are the bindings?
> What behooves us?
> —Adrienne Rich, "An Atlas of the Difficult World"

> Step lightly   all around us
> words are cracking
> off we drift
> separate and syllabic
> if we survive at all
> —Audre Lorde, "Thaw"

In ways strikingly similar to those of Bambara, Marshall, and Naylor, Leslie Marmon Silko treats the issue of individual and collective illness in *Ceremony*, weaving together the narrative of an ailing World War II veteran of mixed-blood heritage with traditional Laguna myth and the tale of a land and society in need of healing.[1] *Ceremony* draws on Native American beliefs (especially Silko's own Laguna traditions) about the interconnectedness of all creation—of human beings with one another and with the rest of the physical world. Silko complicates those interconnections in unmasking the effects of racism and colonization on the illness of her main character, Tayo. In addition, she demonstrates the persistence and complexity of Tayo's resistance to oppression. Indeed, the novel is a record and representation of resistance to what Alan Wald calls "internal colonialism," a state of being that, unacknowledged, complicates the experience of members of "internal colonies" in the United States, such as Native Americans,[2] and what Gloria Anzaldúa calls "internalized dominance."[3] Among other things, *Ceremony* challenges an individualistic worldview that maintains the fiction of self-determination and ignores such social factors as privilege based on race, class, gender, and sexual orientation, factors that underwrite a person's or group's status and power in the world. In this view, those who are marginalized and oppressed by society are left with (and accused of) the devastating sense that the reasons for such exclusion and oppression have more to do with individual personal failings than with social patterns and racist institutional structures. Silko actively interrogates such individualistic thinking. She does this by anatomizing Tayo's illness, situating it in the broader social context of war, racism, and colonialism. While Toni Flores observes that "in Tayo there is a coming together of the sicknesses of the land, nature, the social order, power relations, the family, and the soul,"[4] it is too easy to read this as an indictment of *Tayo's* community and culture, rather than of the unjust structures in which that community is embedded.

The novel also complicates or thickens the idea of a unitary, all-or-nothing resistance, showing how resistance and the experience of domination in fact coexist, and that resistance to domination can take myriad forms, many of which are invisible to those in dominance. Thus, even while Tayo is under the thrall of his illness and of dominant structures of thought and control, at the same time he also resists them. Tayo's empowered stance at the end of the novel against genocide, while an act of profound resistance, is preceded and supported by many less visible acts of resistance that occur throughout the narrative. The novel probes the relationship of resistance to healing, as well as the characteristics of that resistance itself. In *Ceremony*, Tayo's acts of resistance fuel his healing, and in the final analysis, this becomes the primary agent for the maintenance of Tayo's health. The resistance Tayo comes to internalize grows out of the integration that is both sign and substance of his healing. "The purpose of a ceremony is to integrate," says Paula Gunn Allen, "to fuse the individual with his or her fellows, the community of people with that of the other kingdoms, and this larger communal group with the worlds beyond this one."[5]

In many instances, Tayo's small and large acts of resistance themselves call into question the ability of medicine (and the dominant culture in which it is embedded) to interpret and identify health when it presents itself. What appears to be a nervous breakdown on the battlefield, for example, is the result of a profound (and troubling) knowing. In going "crazy," Tayo manifests serious and painful internal distress, but moreover, in so doing, he refuses to submit to the military's definition of the enemy. The doctors who treat Tayo are incapable of interpreting Tayo's distress as anything but the manifestation of pathology. Thus, the novel also raises questions about the ability of an institution primarily composed of members of the dominant class (and primarily serving that class) to interpret and read signs of illness and health in nondominant persons. What appears to be pathology, Silko insists, may indeed be a sign of resistance and itself a marker of health.

Silko also goes beyond representing resistance thematically, creating a text that, in its structure and style, resists readers' expectations of the novelistic narrative form. The text challenges readers to rethink not only what but *how* they read, a criteria bell hooks applies to all "critical fictions." This type of text, she argues, seeks "to deconstruct conventional ways of knowing" and "critically intervenes and challenges dominant/hegemonic narratives by compelling audiences to actually transform the way they read and think."[6] Throughout the novel, chronology is fractured as present folds easily into past and future, and Tayo's perceptions break spatial and temporal barriers. Silko weaves poems and legends throughout the narrative of Tayo's brokenness (a result of his experience both in World War II and in the domestic "war" of racism back home). Silko employs, for example, the story of Reed Woman, Corn Woman, Hummingbird, Fly, and Buzzard, who must discover within themselves ingenuity, interdependence, and perseverance to restore balance to a devastated land and people during a season of drought.[7] Mary Slowik argues that in *Ceremony*, the juxtaposition of what she calls the mythopoetic with narrative creates a "contrapuntal reading" where narrative exists as a fluid form that constructs characters who "are no longer autonomous, self-contained psychological units" but who "can slide into and out of their ancestors, or move easily between the magic and the real."[8]

Resistance is also part of *Ceremony*'s structure as the text brings together the seemingly disparate elements of factual history and myth so that both become part of the same cloth: *Ceremony* is a text that re-members, rejoins, sundered elements. Distinctions between "magic" and "real" are finally unimportant to the complex truths of the story. Similarly, the boundaries between psychosomatic and "real" biomedical disorders and even between the world's body and the body's world become blurred. In *Ceremony*, the illness of Tayo's body and mind is—in the way of an intricate spider web—inextricably bound to social pathologies such as racism, the politics of containment and repression of Native Americans, merciless capitalism, and the unthinking pillage of the earth's body. In the same way that the myth of Hummingbird's rescue of the starving community is part of the narrative of Tayo's return home, Tayo's story is also part of a broad web of meaning that extends far beyond his own individual life. Indeed, the novel complicates the terms of human existence by insisting that distinctions such as "individual" and "community" are, finally, social markers but never ontological realities. Much as individual filaments that connect a web also constitute that web, so Tayo learns that he is both individual and community, but that without the community, his individuality leads to alienation and brokenness.

What such a construction of narrative and character suggests goes counter to the doctors' definitions of mental health. Silko contests the implicit belief that psychological health is embodied only in humans who have clearly defined and well-maintained, individualistic boundaries. But she also problematizes it. If Tayo is to resist dominant ideas about his personhood and his relationship to community, he must negotiate a relationship of resistance to the dominant community, with its dis-membering function, and rejoin himself to a healthy or health-giving community, one that is a community of re-membering. Silko's text argues that the individual, autonomous self is a fiction that furthers the illusion of an ultimately dis-membering individualism at the expense of those who do (for they are deceived) and those who do not fit the dominant norm (and are frequently pronounced sick).

Constructing a central character that is male rather than female, the novel also rewrites the terms of gender difference. By juxtaposing Tayo's illness against his drinking buddies' machismo and callous disregard of the trauma of war, and by associating them with what Silko calls the witchery and its destructive powers,[9] the novel casts one element of Tayo's healing as a reformulating of rigid and dehumanizing gender distinctions. While part of Tayo's healing happens as a result of time spent with medicine men, he is also profoundly influenced and guided by women. The beginning of his journey toward health comes about as a result of his grandmother's loving ministrations. In addition, the remarkable healer Ts'eh, whom Lisa Orr describes as "a woman of the old ways who understands the natural world around her and practices the rituals that enable her to maintain her connection with the earth,"[10] effectively mentors him in the ways of herbal medicine and living on the earth. Allen points out that a significant aspect of Tayo's healing, in fact, is to encounter the mother in himself, in the earth, and in other men and women. Orr claims that a major factor in Tayo's healing is his incorporation of the feminine within himself. However, rather than "feminizing" Tayo, I think instead that Silko unmoors gender from oppositional poles and insists that the distinctions themselves are part of the witchery and make possible atrocities like the war from which Tayo has just returned.[11]

Sickness is not simply a matter of individual biopathology but is necessarily a symptom of larger phenomena. Tayo suffers the effects of having fought a devastating war on two fronts: that of the declared enemy and that of the domestic, always present (but harder to discern) enemy, racism. Tayo therefore not only fights alongside white soldiers but simultaneously has to fight against the annihilating racism they embody. Further, Tayo returns from the war to a world whose dominant powers have historically and actively sought to erase his culture and heritage. Tayo's healing journey is, in many respects, a journey back to himself through story, not unlike that of Velma, Avey, and Ciel. In what bell hooks calls "a struggle of memory against forgetting," Tayo will learn that "remembering makes us subjects in history" and that it is nothing short of "dangerous to forget."[12] In *Ceremony*, however, it is also dangerous to remember, because Tayo's knowledge or memory of who he is makes it impossible for him fully to assimilate into white society with its individualistic constructs of health and well-being. Because of this, he is therefore deemed sick.

Further, since he had a white father, Tayo exists within a liminal space where he is neither Indian nor white. Patricia Riley, drawing on Orval Looking Horse's definition, points out that the Laguna word for a mixed-blood person is *iyeska*, a term that "embodies the concept of one who not only interprets between the red and white worlds, but between the world of spirits and human beings as well."[13] Thus, the pain is also potentially the gift. Anzaldúa writes about borderland space, in her analysis of Chicana women's experience, as the place inhabited by mestizas, women with "mixed blood," like Tayo, who inhabit that space "where the Third World grates up against the first and bleeds." This is also a space, however, of "constant transition."[14] Part of Tayo's healing involves creating or transforming— with the help of the healer Betonie and the others who are part of the extended ceremony—the bleeding borderland space into one that is life giving. As Tayo embarks on the journey of healing with those stronger than he, he weaves together the broken, dis-membered strands of the narrative. While cultural memory makes it possible for him to resist the dominant norms, he still must learn to know *that* he knows and *what* he knows. In so doing, Tayo comes to inhabit that transforming, healing borderland within himself where he is re-membered both within himself and to his community.[15]

Silko, in fact, figures dis-membering as a primary function of what she terms the witchery. Counter to the humanizing and empowering task of re-membering, the witchery dis-members human beings, turning them into bodies without connection or memory. One of the myth-poems in *Ceremony* graphically describes the witches cooking sundered parts of human bodies:

dead babies simmering in blood
circles of skull cut away
all the brains sucked out . . . skin bundles
Whorls of skin
cut from fingertips
sliced from the penis end and clitoris tip. [134]

The witchery, in its ability to fragment human experience (much as the bodies are fragmented in the cook pot), cuts human beings off from themselves, from what they know—even if only in dim memory—about being human. The dismembering employed by the witches and figured as fragmented bodies represents Tayo's confused mental state. Riley explains that "Silko uses the story of the 'witchery' to point out that *how* this counterforce came into existence is not the most important thing. What must be acknowledged is the fact that it does exist and that it will manipulate anyone who allows it to do so."[16]

The cure for witchery, the novel suggests, is to be found in resisting the deadening stories of domination and conquest. Moreover, the cure will be found in retelling the old stories as well as in creating and telling new ones, recasting and reclaiming experience and history that have been warped in such a way that makes domination possible, as one of the storytellers insists at the beginning of the novel:[17]

I will tell you something about stories,
[he said]
They aren't just entertainment.
Don't be fooled.
They are all we have, you see,
all we have to fight off
illness and death.

. . . .
Their evil is mighty
but it can't stand up to our stories.
So they try to destroy the stories
let the stories be confused or forgotten. [2]

Tayo must learn how to rewrite the story created for him and his people by the witchery and its tools: the greed and power of colonizers and the ongoing effects of racism. His task is no less than a rewriting of history— one written long ago in the conquest of the Americas. Tayo's rewritten story will constitute a resistance to colonialism's oppressive effects.[18] In *Ceremony*, medicine's intensification of the colonialist script occurs as doctors actively steer Tayo away from Indian medicine, insisting that he avoid traditional healers, among other things. Tayo's resistance and his healing become a counternarrative to that of Western medicine.

Calling *Ceremony* "a stern and superior criticism of Western medicine and values," B. A. St. Andrews notes that in the novel, "white" medicine "traditionally explores individuality as a healing center, [and] simply misunderstands 'red' philosophy which holds 'the People' as the center and the individual as its radius."[19] There is even more at stake than St. Andrews claims, however. The doctors do not simply "misunderstand"; like the society in which they function, they make no attempt to understand. Instead, they simply disregard Tayo's truths and realities as those of a safely distanced Other. One of the noticeable aspects of white doctoring in *Ceremony* is the explicit disavowal of anything useful outside the bounds of Western biomedicine, as well as the prevailing social climate of privilege (and legitimization) of values and knowledge arising from Euro-American culture alone. In Silko's hands, medicine, like religion (and many other institutions of Euro-American social life), is clearly implicated in oppression. The cure medicine offers is part of a much larger evil that would prompt Tayo to act alone as an autonomous individual, erasing collective and empowering tribal beliefs and traditions. It is witchery that maintains the illusion of self-determination and individualism that so permeates contemporary society. Internalized racism leads Tayo to mistrust his perceptions, feelings, and knowledge, and this prevents his experience of connection; but the internalization is incomplete. Through long struggle and the help of others, Tayo learns why he has insisted on saying "we" and "us" in the white hospital and comes to see how he has resisted all along. Not only will he find healing for (and within) himself, but he will be able to get on with work of collective world healing, resisting and reversing the witchery's effects.

Tayo's story is not far fetched. Mary Crow Dog's autobiography, *Lakota Woman*, vividly captures the alienating effects of colonization and examines how her encounters with the white world inevitably resulted in attempts to erase her Native culture and roots. She remembers that Catholic missionaries were famous for telling the Indians that they "*must kill the Indian in order to save the man.*"[20] Crow Dog's observations about, and experiences in, the government-mandated boarding schools underscore the concrete ways government and religious institutions attempted to "save the man":

> The schools were intended as an alternative to the outright
> extermination seriously advocated by generals Sherman
> and Sheridan, as well as by most settlers and prospectors
> over-running our land. "You don't have to kill those poor
> benighted heathen," the do-gooders said, "in order to solve
> the Indian Problem. Just give us a chance to turn them into
> useful farmhands, laborers, and chambermaids who will
> break their backs for you at low wages." In that way the
> boarding schools were born. The kids were taken away
> from their villages and pueblos, in their blankets and moc-
> casins, kept completely isolated from their families—
> sometimes for as long as ten years—suddenly coming
> back, their short hair slick with pomade, their necks raw
> from stiff, high collars . . . caricatures of white people.[21]

Crow Dog also cites a set of rules, a "ten commandments" for colonized Indians, given to her grandfather by missionaries for him to display on his wall (and which she still possesses). These rules are stunning in their blatant disregard for Native American ways and their unselfconscious championing of the civic gospel of what Crow Dog calls "whitemanization," as well as for their paternalistic and infantilizing dictates: "Come out of your blanket, cut your hair, and dress like a white man"; "Live in a house like your white brother. Work hard and wash often"; "Speak the language of your white brother."[22]

Take Tayo's Auntie, for example. The external racism and coercion that Crow Dog describes leads to the kind of shame and ambivalence that Tayo's Auntie feels about herself and her family. Unlike Tayo, she has left no openings within herself for possible resistance. As a child, Tayo experienced Auntie's hard shell when, at age four, he was left by his alcoholic mother to live with her and her family. His aunt takes him in "to conceal the shame of her younger sister" (29) but treats him always as an outsider, afraid of guilt by association in the eyes of the white world. Born to a woman who could not care for him and a white man he never saw, Tayo lives in uneasy tension with Auntie, who uses Christianity as a bludgeon to punish Tayo for his mother's transgressions. The narrator tells the disturbing story of Tayo attempting to survive in trash heaps of the arroyo where he, his mother, and the other homeless of Gallup lived in cardboard shacks: "When she woke up at noon she would call the child to bring her water. The lard pail was almost empty; the water looked rusty. He waited until she crawled to the opening. He watched her throat moving up and down as she drank; he tried to look inside to see if she had brought food. . . . She dropped the pail when it was empty and crawled back inside. 'Muh!' he called to her because he was hungry and he had found no food that morning" (109).

Displacing her rage at Tayo's mother and her own self-hatred onto Tayo, Auntie sees in him all that she believes degrading about being Indian (and is perhaps afraid of the quiet resistance to her way of life that she senses in him). She thus shuts him out emotionally while caring for him physically. Auntie's rigid Christianity disavows any connection with Native American spirituality or customs. ("Christianity separated the people from themselves . . . encouraging each person to stand alone," claims the narrator [68]). The narrator suggests, in fact, that Christianity is a powerful agent in the downfall of Tayo's mother and that Auntie might have helped "little sister" had Auntie not disavowed Indian ways.

Much as Christianity has functioned as an alienating factor in Tayo's family life, so, too, has medicine. Having treated his malaria and having tried (but failed) to treat what they deem to be psychotic symptoms related to the trauma of battle, the physicians at the Veterans Administration discharge Tayo. "No Indian medicine," they warn him, admitting at the same time that the causes of Tayo's diagnosed battle fatigue are "a mystery, even to them" (31). As part of their post-hospitalization advice, the doctors have told Tayo "that he had to think only of himself and not about the others, that he would never get well as long as he used words like 'we' and 'us'" (125). Leaving the hospital in a daze, Tayo notices the cardboard name tag on his suitcase and realizes that "it had been a long time since he had thought about having a name" (16).

Ceremony's implicit critique of oppressive medical practice also implies a challenge: can medicine, in Adrienne Rich's words about Jewish feminists, turn "Otherness into a keen lens of empathy, that we can bring into being a politics based on concrete, heartfelt understanding of what it means to be Other"?[23] While many medical schools teach "biopsychosocial" concepts of medical practice and have added ethics and interdisciplinary courses to their curricula, and while several psychiatrists bring the practice of "witness" to their interactions with patients, there is much distance between the mere recognition of Otherness and the use of it as a "lens of empathy." *Ceremony* suggests that it is within the context of specific, culturally based community that healing is catalyzed. This does not rule out medical intervention, but it does indicate that medicine will not always be the final arbiter in healing.

Indeed, Tayo leaves the hospital as sick as or sicker than when he entered, excruciatingly nauseated, disoriented, feverish, and haunted by nightmares of his recent war experience. Tayo's story makes clear, as Arthur Frank argues, that certain "bodily symptoms are the infolding of cultural traumas into the body."[24] Similar to Avey's illness in *Praisesong for the Widow*, Tayo's symptoms are often vague and include a swelling in his belly, "a great swollen grief that was pushing into his throat" (9). Stomach "shivering" and knotted like the tangled spools of thread he had played with as a child, Tayo is practically immobilized by his chronic vomiting, fatigue, and a depression that keeps him almost continually weeping. Without diminishing the pain he feels, however, it is important to read in Tayo's physical signs what Scott calls "hidden transcripts of resistance." Arthur Kleinman, studying resistance in patients with chronic pain, notes that in its "usual sense," resistance is employed against "the imposition of dominating definitions (diagnoses), norms defining how we should behave (prescriptions), and official accounts (records) of what had happened." Kleinman describes finding a kind of resistance that "comes from bodily forms of expressing political alienation and resistance to the powers of authority."[25] Tayo's body itself turns away from dominant medicine, causing him to seek a more authentic healing journey within the Native community.

Ceremony throws into bold relief medicine's limited understanding of the context and function of Tayo's illness as well as its limited resources to deal with him. The doctors insist that Tayo repudiate his tribal loyalties, repudiate the knowledge he already has, but in his own mind has neither fully understood nor legitimized. They urge him to treat himself as an isolated—somehow autonomous—individual, advice that undermines the requirement of the Hippocratic Oath to "do no harm." It is as if Tayo were in the position of Africans in the late nineteenth century who "were expected to participate in their colonization by silencing their own sociocultural histories," writes Sally Swartz in her study of insanity in the Cape Colony. She points out Megan Vaughan's observation that "it was the colonial subjects who were insufficiently Other, who had 'forgotten' who they were [as subjects], and had ceased to conform to the notion of the African subject, who most often found themselves behind the walls of the asylum."[26] Given the lens through which medicine sees (or does not see) Tayo and assesses his illness, it is not surprising that Tayo senses that he is nothing but "white smoke" that "had no consciousness of itself" (14). He recalls that "their medicine drained memory out of his thin arms and replaced it with a twilight cloud behind his eyes" (15). The whiteness with which Tayo is surrounded in the hospital—the walls, sheets, and uniforms— mirrors the anni-hilating, erasing whiteness of the dominant culture, turning him into "invisible scattered smoke" (14). Those things the doctors tell Tayo and try to force him to accept are the very things that will create the invisibility he experiences.[27]

Silko's use of invisibility as a trope recalls Ralph Ellison's, how-ever. Like the Invisible Man of Ellison's novel, Tayo becomes in-visible as a result of white ignorance and racism, but also like the Invisible Man, Tayo uses that invisibility strategically. As "smoke," Tayo cannot be controlled, contained, or manipulated.[28] (In addition, the image of smoke brings to mind the way smoke signals were used by various Native American tribes as ways of communication, warn-ings to those equipped to recognize them.) Tayo speaks of himself to the hospital psychiatrist in the distancing form of the third person, refusing the psychiatrist access: "He can't talk to you. He is invisible. His words are formed with an invisible tongue, they have no sound" (15). Tayo knows (but again, is not quite sure that he knows) that not only do the doctors not enable his healing, but they maintain and exacerbate his illness. Aída Hurtado discusses the use of silence as "a powerful weapon when it can be controlled. It is akin to camouflag-ing oneself when at war in an open field, playing possum at strategic times causes the power of the silent one to be underestimated."[29]

When one psychiatrist does finally break through Tayo's resis-tance enough to cause him to cry, Tayo briefly abandons the third person and says, "Goddam you . . . look what you have done" (16). The scene in the hospital is complicated, however. While Tayo's distance from the doctors is a sign of resistance, he is also in danger of existing in the state that is the witchery's highest goal: as a nonfeeling human being who cannot even cry, "not even for yourself" (229). The doctor pushes Tayo into feeling something as a means of thera-peutic intervention, using Silko's own criteria for gauging the damage of the witchery. It is unfair, I believe, to call the Veterans Administra-tion hospital "a house of bad medicine staffed with witch doctors," as one critic has done.[30] Silko creates a hospital that is clearly as much captive to the witchery as the other institutions and society within which it is situated. But even in this place where Tayo cannot become well, there is a moment in which he is called out of a resistance that could become damaging, and into feeling. The problem is that without the context of story and community, Tayo's tears would remain tears of impotent rage. The hospital scenes in *Ceremony* suggest that medicine has its limits and that while therapeutic intervention may be helpful to a point, one must go further. In this instance, the doctors attempt to block a therapeutic move away from medicine and into another means of healing. They also disallow Tayo his own story.

What the doctors do not know and have not begun to find out is that, along with the malaria, battle fatigue, and hallucinations they have correctly diagnosed, Tayo is also wracked with grief about the untimely death (and his failure to prevent it) of his beloved cousin, Rocky, as they fought alongside each other in Korea. He also grieves for his Uncle Josiah (with whom Tayo had worked and planned to work after the war), who died at home during Tayo's absence. Once he has returned home from the hospital, Tayo is barely able to leave his bed and feels "there [is] no place left for him; [that] he would find no peace in that house where silence and the emptiness echoed the loss" (32).

Begrudgingly cared for by his aunt, Tayo has become "tired of fighting off the dreams and the voices . . . tired of guarding himself against places and things which evoked his memories" (26). After weeks of no improvement, in desperation and loneliness Tayo calls out to his grandmother for help. She is the antithesis of what the white doctors have advised: an old blind Indian woman.

> His voice was shaking; he called her. He wanted to tell her
> they had to take him back to the hospital. He watched her
> get up slowly, with old bones that were stems of thin glass
> she shuffled across the linoleum in her cloth slippers, mov-
> ing cautiously as if she did not trust memory to take her to

his bed. She sat down on the edge of the bed and she
reached out for him. She held his head in her lap and she
cried with him, saying "A'moo'oh, a'moo'ohh" over and
over again. [33]

Similar to the kind of touch that occurs in *Praisesong for the Widow*,
The Women of Brewster Place, and *The Salt Eaters*, this physical contact and release marks an important moment in Tayo's resistance and
healing. Edith Swan points out that, unlike Tayo's aunt, "Grandma is
traditional, bearing her Laguna heritage with pride. . . . She is convinced of the dignity and efficacious nature of tribal methods for
curing and sanity—precepts undergirding her insistence that medicine men (Ku'oosh and Betonie) treat her grandson Tayo."[31] The
moments in his grandmother's arms mark the beginning of an intentional recasting, a healing, of his past relationships with absent or
disapproving mother figures as his tears intermingle with hers, signifying both a cleansing process and a human, collective connection
that will lead him toward health. "Those white doctors haven't helped
you at all" (33), his grandmother croons, providing the most accurate
diagnosis so far. Tayo listens to his grandmother, and her words
resonate with his own knowledge, delegitimized though it is by the
dominant culture, especially by medicine.

   To his white-identified Auntie's dismay, Tayo's grandmother sends
for the local medicine man, Ku'oosh: "He spoke softly, using the old
dialect full of sentences that were involuted with explanations of
their own origins, as if nothing the old man said were his own but all
had been said before and he was only there to repeat it" (34). Ku'oosh
acknowledges "the distant circumstance of [Tayo's] absent white father" and points to the possibility that there are things Tayo does not
know (connected to his being an Indian) that perhaps Josiah (Tayo's
uncle) might have taught him "before [Tayo] went to the white people's big war." Addressing Tayo as "grandson," Ku'oosh tells him "this
world is fragile" (35) as a sun-shot spider web, and that even one
person could "tear away the delicate strands of the web, spilling the
rays of the sun into the sand," injuring the entire world (38). Listen-

ing to Ku'oosh, Tayo moves closer to what he has known all along but that has been blurred and obscured as he has walked the potentially dangerous path between the Indian and non-Indian worlds. Specifically, he begins to re-member, to strengthen the ligaments of knowing (the strands of the web) as he ponders the meaning of community, the responsibility of personhood.

Ku'oosh pointedly asks Tayo about the possibility that he may have killed or touched a dead person and therefore defiled (and sickened) himself. Ku'oosh admits to Tayo that "there are some things we can't cure like we used to" (38). War, with its machines that allow men to kill one another without even seeing or knowing that killing has occurred, calls for ceremonies different from those used in the past. Ku'oosh knows that Tayo and the other reservation war veterans will need a new ceremony to deal with the technologies of modern war. Other veterans on the reservation had undergone the scalp ceremony (where the scalp of warriors is ritually nicked to protect them against being haunted by those they had killed or touched), but they had ended up no better for it, laments Ku'oosh. (Tayo wonders about this, though, since they seem not to feel things as he does and thus, to him, appear much stronger than he.) Silko's narrator reminds readers, though, that the witchery's "highest ambition is to gut human beings while they are still breathing, to hold the heart still beating so the victim will never feel anything again" (229). Harley, Pinkie, and Emo want nothing more than to remember the "power" they felt in uniform, and they drink alcohol to forget that their power never existed in the first place.[32] Alcohol is one instrument that performs the gutting function for the witchery. While Tayo's sensitivity to the insanity of war makes him ill, his insight contains within it the seeds of his healing. Tayo feels and responds; his friends do not.

The Indian tea and blue cornmeal Ku'oosh leaves with Tayo help heal his physical symptoms (he vomits less and sleeps more soundly). But Tayo remains visibly ill, prompting the tribal council to send him to Old Betonie, a Navajo healer (of mixed blood, like Tayo—"My grandmother was a remarkable Mexican with green eyes," he declares [119]). Betonie's dwelling is north of the Gallup ceremonial grounds and overlooks the site where Tayo had lived in squalor and precarious survival as a baby. It is here that the ceremony evolves to meet the moment, to deal with the complicated effects of war, colonization, and internal racism—and Tayo's entrapment in the witchery.

Betonie's house appears to Tayo as a chaotic collection of odds and ends and the product of an even more chaotic mind. As he becomes accustomed to the dim light, however, he slowly realizes there is a pattern to the "boxes and trunks, the bundles and stacks [that] . . . followed the concentric shadows of the room" (120). Tayo's realization of the patterns in this circular house built in the side of a hill with a sky hole in the middle mirrors his growing awareness of the patterns in his own life. For Tayo, assimilation has meant viewing his life and culture through the eyes of white domination, and his vision is thus distorted to the extent that he fails to see the pattern of truth underneath the chaotic lies. Like Betonie's home, Tayo's life appears to be radically Other to him until—in the process of healing—he begins to reclaim it by perceiving it through a different lens. Tayo views Betonie's hogan as though he is two people (as though the son of the white man and the son of the Indian woman were at odds with each other), "deceived by the poverty he sees in Betonie's hogan, looking for that moment through the eyes of the colonized at what has been 'lost,' and through the eyes of the colonizer at what he reads as a material lack."[33] To Tayo,

> all of it seemed suddenly so pitiful and small compared to the world he knew the white people had—a world of comfort in the sprawling houses he'd seen in California, a world of plenty in the food he had carried from the officers' mess to dump into garbage cans. The old man's clothes were dirty and old, probably collected like his calendars. The leftover things the whites didn't want. All Betonie owned in the world was in this room. What kind of healing power was in this? [127]

Indeed, *Ceremony* radically displaces the locus of healing. Not in the hospital or medical technologies, but in this place furnished with the discards of white people, this poor house with all its precarious possessions, in Betonie's wisdom and the force of the story he and Tayo unfold, does healing power reside.

What does it mean that the discards of the white people form a pattern? Or that the pattern itself contained healing power? The truths Tayo sees in those scraps and the apparent chaos are no less than the truths embodied in the ways of seeing that make the space for the counternarrative Tayo and Betonie create together. They have to work at creating this narrative, however. The pull of a dominant worldview is hard to resist. Invisibility and white medicine (like alcohol), as a means to kill the pain, is seductive. Questioning Betonie about the fact that he had not felt any pain at the white hospital, Tayo wonders if perhaps he belongs back there. Betonie counters by suggesting that Tayo would be better off drinking himself to death than returning to the white man's hospital, likening modern psychiatric treatment to a slow death for people of color: "You might as well go down there [to the arroyo], with the rest of them, sleeping in the mud, vomiting cheap wine, rolling over women. Die that way and get it over with. . . . In that hospital they don't bury the dead, they keep them in rooms and talk to them" (123).

With Betonie, Tayo chooses to resist a living death, realizing that he had known all along that the doctors were wrong, even as he was trying to believe their admonition to "think only of himself, and not about the others." Tayo knows that real healing, real medicine "didn't work that way, because the world didn't work that way" (125). Tayo realizes that "his sickness was only part of something larger, and his cure would be found only in something great and inclusive of everything" (125–26). Thus Tayo's healing becomes a process of recognizing and repudiating the colonized state of mind that would accept the doctor's views without question.

Frantz Fanon's analysis of the process of decolonization points to the function of individualism that Tayo's doctors had insisted on.

Individualism is the first to disappear. The native intellectual had learnt from his masters that the individual ought
to express himself fully. The colonialist bourgeoisie had
hammered into the native's mind the idea of a society of
individuals where each person shuts himself up in his own
subjectivity, and whose only wealth is individual thought.
Now the native who has the opportunity to return to the
people during the struggle for freedom will discover the
falseness of this theory. . . . Henceforward, the interests of
one will be the interests of all, for in concrete fact *everyone*
will be discovered by the troops, *everyone* will be
massacred—or *everyone* will be saved.[34]

For Tayo, white medicine, especially white psychiatric medicine, is
equated with nothing short of destruction, and his move away from it
represents his own liberatory process. Medicine, as Betonie portrays
it, is a culturally and emotionally anesthetizing and alienating practice, consigning people to a living death. In *Ceremony*, medicine, like
Fanon's colonialist bourgeoisie, maintains the theory and practice of
a dis-membering individualism.

A central question for Tayo is whether he will trust himself and
his own knowledge, assessment, and critique of his world. Together
he and Betonie construct a re-membered story, a narrative that counters the colonized script against which Tayo has been struggling.
Their act of restor(y)ing powerfully resists the witchery. In telling his
story, Tayo finds the strength to question and critique a system that
accords value on the basis of skin color, even though in war Tayo had
seen that the skin of his white corporal "was not much different from
his own" (7). This insight into the insanity of racism, however, rather
than empowering Tayo, had increased his sense of alienation and self-
doubt because he had no story, no narrative context that supported
such an observation while he was in the war and later, while he was
struggling in the hospital.

Indeed, as the boundaries of difference based on skin and ethnicity begin to blur, killing becomes impossible for Tayo. For him,

"the worst thing" is that the racial otherness he had learned in the United States no longer buttresses his military obedience, since even his enemies "looked too familiar . . . when they were alive" (7). Once otherness collapses, as it does for Tayo, war becomes the ultimate insanity. Tayo thus embodies the only sane response to war: to go crazy. Rather than trusting his perceptions as accurate critique, Tayo and, of course, those around him suppose that he is insane and has simply lost his mind to battle fatigue. Because of what he knows, because of the traces of collectivity he retains, Tayo is unable to accept the notion of otherness that permits indiscriminate killing, and this marks him as a sick man.

For example, when Tayo's commanding officer orders him to pull the trigger and kill Japanese prisoners, Tayo freezes because he sees in one of them the face of his Uncle Josiah.

> So Tayo stood there, stiff with nausea, while they fired at
> the soldiers, and he watched his uncle fall, and he *knew* it
> was Josiah; and even after Rocky started shaking him by
> the shoulders and telling him to stop crying, it was *still*
> Josiah lying there. They forced medicine into Tayo's
> mouth, and Rocky pushed him toward the corpses and told
> him to look. . . . "Look, Tayo, look at the face," and that was
> when Tayo started screaming. [8; emphasis in original]

Because he has been so completely separated from any nourishing ground, Tayo becomes sick. Moreover, his real problem is that he simply cannot tolerate war's insanity and, in fact, sees no difference between his skin and Japanese skin; thus he sees through the artificial distinctions war imposes (*enemies, them, us*).[35] A medic is summoned, and "the next day they all acted as though nothing had happened," calling Tayo's collapse battle fatigue and hallucinations connected to malarial fever (8).

While facts and logic fail to help Tayo construct an explanatory framework for his war experience, his breakdown signals another form of resistance, masked though it may be by medically defined

symptoms. Rocky had tried to explain to Tayo that while he understands his "homesickness," Tayo should realize that "we're *supposed*
to be here. This [killing] is what we're supposed to do" (8). Tayo's
inability to do the work of war makes him, in the eyes of the rest of
the world, crazy. With Betonie, however, Tayo's perceptions (and his
implicit agency) are confirmed and given an etiology: "It isn't surprising," Betonie tells him, that "you saw [Josiah] with them. You saw
who they were. Thirty thousand years ago they were not strangers.
You saw what the evil had done: you saw the witchery ranging as
wide as this world" (124). Tayo's breakdown is actually a breakout,
or a break away from the lies that are perpetuated by the military and
state apparatus to which he is subject. While the doctors see Tayo's
symptoms as pathology to medicate and treat, the novel suggests
otherwise, foregrounding the function of counternarratives such as
that created by Betonie and Tayo as empowering agents of understanding and healing.

Another of Tayo's ravaging memories has to do with the circumstances surrounding the death of Rocky, his cousin (and Auntie's
son). Having been swept into enlisting by Rocky's enthusiasm
(Rocky calls Tayo "brother" for the first time) and the vision of living
and fighting side by side with him, Tayo feels not only the loss of
Rocky but the guilt of knowing that of the two, the "wrong one" had
been killed. Tayo has known all along that Rocky was the chosen, the
one who would go to college, who "understood what he had to do to
win in the white outside world." "He was an A-student and all-state in
football and track. He had to win; he said he was always going to win.
So he listened to his teachers, and he listened to the coach. They were
proud of him. They told him, 'Nothing can stop you now except one
thing: don't let the people at home hold you back'" (51). While
Rocky is the named hero and chooses the right/white way, Tayo is
actually the winner, standing not only as a hero by the end of the
novel but as one who is still alive. *Ceremony* thus disrupts white-
defined formulas for success. Rocky, following the rules, ends up
losing his life due to heat, torrential rain, and no medical care. After
they are captured by the Japanese, Tayo and his corporal carry Rocky

on the muddy road to the prison camp. Slipping and barely able to breathe in the steaming rain, Tayo prays desperately for dry air, "dry as a hundred years squeezed out of yellow sand, air to dry out the oozing wounds of Rocky's leg, to let the torn flesh and broken bones breathe, to clear the sweat that filled Rocky's eyes" (11). When the blanket on which Tayo and the corporal carry Rocky is ripped loose during a flash flood, Tayo damns the rain "until the words were a chant, and he sang it while he crawled through the mud to find the corporal and get him up before the Japanese saw them" (12). As Tayo has feared, when the Japanese see Rocky's gangrene, they crush his head with a rifle butt. Back home, overcome with guilt and grief, Tayo believes that the current drought has been caused by his curse, that he has "prayed the rain away." He sees himself as an "accident of time and space: Rocky was the one who was alive. . . . It was him, Tayo, who had died, but somehow there had been a mistake with the corpses, and somehow his was still unburied" (28).

Despite Tayo's obvious and intense suffering, Betonie connects his illness with his responsibility to the community: "We've all been waiting for help. . . . But it never has been easy. The people must do it. You must do it" (125). Echoing *The Salt Eaters'* Minnie Ransom insisting that there is "weight" to being well, Betonie makes it clear that Tayo's illness is connected to a larger dynamic. Healing will demand a certain volition and participation on his part—not the individualistic and alienating volition that the white doctors call for, but a willingness to move further into the ceremony's pattern and to rediscover his part in, and the strands that connect him to, the larger web of the human community.

Betonie warns Tayo against hating all whites (including himself as a mixed blood), giving him a clearheaded (and nonessentialist) view of human nature: "You don't write off all the white people, just like you don't trust all the Indians" (128). In addition, Betonie tells Tayo "his cure would be found only in something great and inclusive of everything" (126). Tayo, then, not only undergoes the ceremonies for himself, but he learns them to use among his people. Despite wondering "what good Indian ceremonies can do against the sickness which comes from [white] wars, [white] bombs, [white] lies" (132), Tayo listens to Betonie. His cure resides in the potentially liberating borderland that Tayo as a mixed blood physically embodies. This is not to say that Tayo necessarily carries mystical properties for healing within himself, but Silko has inscribed in Tayo's physical characteristics a resistance to destructive and essentialist dichotomies ("white" or "Indian") and insists that healing will evolve in part by breaking out of such narrow and socially constructed markers. These same markers and others like them allow for the atrocities of war and its aftermath in the lives of individuals and communities, this novel suggests.

Neither fully belonging to the Native American community nor fully outside it, Tayo is akin to the child Betonie tells him about who goes to live with bears and becomes so alienated from humans that he has to be called back into the community "step by step," so that he would not be in-between forever. "I will bring you back," chants the storyteller,

> Following my footprints
> walk home
> following my footprints
> Come home, happily
> return belonging to your home [143].

It is what William Bevis would call a "homing in," a process common to Native American novels where the hero "regress[ing] to a place, a past where one has been before, is not only the primary story, it is a primary mode of knowledge and a primary good."[36] Betonie teaches Tayo that going "home" cannot occur if an aspect of one's heritage is repudiated. A large part of Tayo's initial healing, however, rests on his being called back into community, being called into who he is.

The novel clearly privileges the Native American community as the place of life affirmation and healing for Tayo, and *Ceremony* does not fail to critique dominant white culture. It is not an essentialist notion of *whiteness* (itself a radically unstable category), however, but the destruction inherent in dominance that the novel critiques. *Ceremony* foregrounds the need to return from alien culture, from that which drains speech, stories, and identities, much as the opening poem of the novel suggests. As Audre Lorde's words warn, "we drift / separate and syllabic / if we survive at all," and we must find the means to join syllables into words, and words into healing stories. Tayo's sense of oneness with creation is revitalizing, devastating, and transcendent, much as his correct recognition of kinship with the Japanese prisoners was both devastating and liberating. As a result of the stories—the counternarratives constructed by Betonie and Tayo, in speech and in ceremony—Tayo realizes that "there were no boundaries; the world below and the sand paintings inside became the same that night" (145).

While the ceremony returns Tayo home to himself and his sense of himself in community, the healing journey also involves action, a literal journey for Tayo mapped by a pattern of stars drawn in the sand by Betonie: "Remember these stars. . . . I've seen them and I've seen the spotted cattle; I've seen a mountain and I've seen a woman" (152). Tayo waits until late September, when he sees the pattern in the North. He sets off in that direction and meets and learns from Ts'eh, a woman who, as Edith Swan, Paula Gunn Allen, and others have pointed out, is a medicine woman and more.[37] Ts'eh, the rainmaker who brings life-giving tears to Tayo (as his grandmother has done), tells him that his Uncle Josiah's wild Mexican cows had been stolen by a white man. Tayo still bears vestiges of internalized racism, expressing doubt that a white man would steal, and realizes that he would never hesitate to accuse a Mexican or an Indian. "He knew then he had learned the lie by heart—the lie which they had wanted him to learn: only brown-skinned people were thieves" (191).

Tayo recovers the cattle; indeed, hunting them is important to his recovery. The acknowledgment that the white men were thieves, his resistance to that thievery, and the growing reliance on Betonie's and Ts'eh's guidance, along with his own sense of being part of a larger pattern, renews and strengthens Tayo. The snows begin to fall—

auguring well for rain—as Tayo herds the cattle through the twenty-foot-long hole he has cut in the white owner's fence. The rupture in the fence and the delivery of cattle from the ranch suggests a birth, with Tayo acting as midwife to justice and his own sense of power and freedom. Tayo's midwifery, however, is characterized by filaments of connection to his community through such people as Betonie, Ts'eh, Tayo's grandmother, and Ku'oosh, those who have witnessed his confusion and pain, and who have helped him move through that pain. Tayo now knows that he functions within a web of connections that makes such bold acts of resistance possible.

Even when he returns to live alone in the remote family ranch house to watch the cattle and sheep, the connections remain and, in fact, are brought to a test. Ts'eh stays with Tayo long enough to teach him more about the roots and plants she gathers, to nurture the growing sense of harmony within him and his connection to healing spiritual forces, and to warn him about the continuing threat to his well-being. The Laguna people, relying on lies told by his enemy Emo, "think you might need the doctors again," explains Ts'eh (228). Indeed, having brought the police and doctors for Tayo and failing to find him (since he heeded the warning), the government people and tribal elders get tired of looking and go home. Emo, Harley, Leroy, and Pinkie, however, remain in the mountains. After long hours of drinking, Emo and Pinkie begin to torture Harley and eventually murder him for letting Tayo get away, as Tayo, hidden from all of them, watches in horror.

Tayo realizes that the place where the torture is occurring is the site the United States had mined for the uranium (1942–45) that was used in the first atomic bomb explosion at Trinity Site, only 300 miles to the southeast at White Sands.[38] The bomb itself was created 100 miles northeast, at Los Alamos. Where Tayo stands, then, and where Harley is tortured is "the point of convergence where the fate of all living things, and even the earth, had been laid" (246).[39] Thus Silko links the social and political evil of witchery with the destruction of the earth's body by the technological apparatus of war (and warfare itself). Tayo knows that what they were doing to Harley "had been intended for [him]" (251), and in this momentous night of the unfolding story, he must struggle against his deep desire to avenge Harley and thus avoid becoming part of the witchery.

> He understood that Harley had bargained for it; he realized that Harley knew how it would end if he failed to get the victim he had named. But Tayo could not endure it any longer. He was certain his own sanity would be destroyed if he did not stop them and all the suffering and dying they caused—the people incinerated and exploded, and little children asleep on streets outside Gallup bars. He was not strong enough to stand by and watch any more. . . . He visualized the contours of Emo's skull; the GI haircut exposed thin bone at the temples, bone that would flex slightly before it gave way under the thrust of the steel edge. [252]

But Tayo knows that "he had only to complete this night, to keep the story out of the reach of the destroyers for a few more hours, and their witchery would turn, upon itself, upon them" (247). Even in an attempt to rescue Harley, Tayo's motives of hatred for Emo would have aligned him with the forces of destruction in which the other three men were caught. It is essential that Tayo stay out of the evil web and therefore change the story's colonialist script that would have Tayo caught in the intratribal violence and self-destruction he sees in his friends.

Embedded in the description of Tayo's moral battle is the story of Hummingbird and Fly attaining the means to purify their town and thereby bring rain to the people: "Here it is. We finally got it but it / sure wasn't very easy" (255). In the context of Tayo's Laocöonian struggle, Hummingbird and Fly offer comic relief. Commenting like a Greek chorus, they remind readers that the business of healing and being healed is *never* easy. After successfully resisting the urge to kill Emo, Tayo returns to the kiva with Ku'oosh and the other old men of his tribe and slowly tells them the story. In the kiva, Tayo undergoes a final cleansing ritual and becomes one of the strong, healed, and healing presences within his community.

Although Silko's notion of witchery has its mystical elements, it is firmly grounded in politically and socially oppressive systems. Silko insists on the responsibility of all people—especially those in dominance— to work toward the dissolution of oppression. For example, the use of alcohol by Tayo and his friends may indeed be a tool of the witchery, but it is effective precisely because it is clearly related to their anger and self-hatred as Indians. "Liquor was medicine . . . medicine for tight bellies and choked-up throats" (40). Harley had boasted, "We got it easy. . . . Nothing for us war heroes to do but lay around and sleep all day" (22). In truth, there *is* little for the men to do, and as the novel suggests, the alcohol consumption renders them harmless to the dominant society during a time of urgent competition for jobs and social position in a postwar era.[40] Although the men have come back in the United States with purple hearts, they find themselves stripped of whatever power they had felt as soldiers; the purple hearts are vacuous deceits.[41] Only the uniform had transformed them into Men; without it, Tayo furiously points out, they are "simply" Indians (and in this assertion lie the seeds of Emo's hatred of Tayo).

> I'm half-breed. I'll be the first to say it. I'll speak for both sides. First time you walked down the street in Gallup or Albuquerque, you knew. Don't lie. You knew right away. The war was over, the uniform was gone. All of a sudden that man at the store waits on you last, makes you wait until all the white people bought what they wanted. And the white lady at the bus depot, she's real careful now not to touch your hand when she counts out your change. [42]

The men hate themselves for losing the feeling of agency they had experienced during the war; "they never talked about it, but they blamed themselves just like they blamed themselves for losing the land the white people took" (43). Unlike Tayo, however, they fully internalize the racism and punish themselves for the effects of the oppressive society into which the white man's war returns them. Anesthetizing the pain robs them of the connection to the meaning of their experience in the war, as well as the necessary energy to resist the self-annihilating impulses. Mary Crow Dog discusses how drinking serves as an accepted form of genocide.

> Supposedly you drink to forget. The trouble is you don't forget, you remember—all the old insults and hatreds, real and imagined. As a result there are always fights. One of the nicest, gentlest men I knew killed his wife in a drunken rage. One uncle had both his eyes put out while he was lying senseless. My sister-in-law Delphine's husband lost one eye. She herself was beaten to death by a drunken tribal policeman. Such things are not even considered worth an investigation [by the government].[42]

In *Ceremony*, Emo and his friends desperately want "to get back that old feeling, that feeling they belonged to America the way they felt during the war" (43), but in Emo's sarcastic boasts, his contempt of Indian ways and ultimately of himself and his place in the United States is evident: "Look what's here for us. Look. Here's the Indians' mother earth! Old dried-up thing!" (25). It is not surprising that by the end of the novel, Harley and Leroy are found dead and, in accord with the witchery's goals, "dismembered beyond recognition" in a crashed pickup truck, "not much different than if they had died at Wake Island or Iwo Jima" (259). Neither is it surprising that Emo later murders Pinkie in a drinking brawl the FBI dismissively calls an accident.

Tayo learns that individualistic health is an impossibility. It is engagement with the world that initiates and helps sustain the restoration of balance.[43] As Tayo trusts his own knowledge, his relief is intense: "He cried the relief he felt at finally seeing the pattern, the way all the stories fit together—the old stories, the war stories, their stories—to become the story that was still being told. He was not crazy; he had never been crazy. He had only seen and heard the world as it always was: no boundaries, only transitions through all distances and time" (246). Throughout his illness the stories have been insistent and have demanded a hearing. Tayo's listening to the wisdom of others and to himself has helped him see patterns and therefore to see the way out of his illness. Silko insists, however, that Tayo's illness can never be separated from the illness of the world, especially the social sickness of racism and genocide in which his doctors wittingly or unwittingly participated.

Does my reading of *Ceremony* leave out medicine altogether? I think not. As I noted earlier in this chapter, other critics have written medicine off. Bonnie Winsbro, for example, argues that the gulf separating Native American and white cultures precludes any positive outcome Tayo might have had in the white hospital "because his illness derives from . . . Laguna Pueblo beliefs [to which Tayo adheres]."[44] In other words, because Tayo's belief system is different from the dominant beliefs, it is a foregone conclusion that medicine would not be able to help him. It seems to me, however, that this notion not only completely dismisses Western medicine; it also lets it too easily off the hook. Healing is rarely a linear, progressive, easily mapped function. And if it does have to depend on a "shared belief system between patient and healer," as Winsbro argues, most of us are in trouble. In Silko's text, medicine has simply not done the necessary work of recognizing its limits in the overall healing process (much larger and more complicated than medicine can deal with alone) or its possibilities (in using otherness as a lens for empathy, e.g.).

Tayo's wisdom in using "we," in reaching back to the traditions and stories of his community, is an essential aspect of his healing, one that is vigorously suppressed by his physicians. Had they been able to listen, however—really listen—they might have found that Tayo held the keys to his healing within him that would have allowed them to help him puzzle out what he needed to do for himself, rather than insisting on drugs and their own therapies based on an individualistic worldview. Arthur Kleinman questions "the practice through which the suffering that is part of a serious medical disorder is reinterpreted as a depressive disease so that an institutionally efficient technical fix (a drug) can be applied in place of a humanely significant relationship of witnessing, affirming, and engaging the patient's and family's existential experience."[45] Such witnessing would likely lead the patient eventually out of the medical setting and into the community for another, different, richer kind of healing, but this, it seems to me, is exactly what a healing intervention should be. Imagine what the physicians would have learned from Tayo's experience. Imagine how much of Tayo's suffering would have been allayed had the doctors simply listened to him. But Silko demands that readers imagine even more. Think what the world would be like without the insane atrocities of war, racism, genocide, and poverty. Perhaps then we can imagine Tayo never having become ill in the first place.

Death Is a Skipped Meal Compared to This

Rememory and the Body in Toni Morrison's *Beloved*

3

How do we get to that promised motherland?
—Marilyn Nelson Waniek, "X Ennead I. Vi"

we will wear
new bones again.
we will leave
these rainy days,
break out through
another mouth
into sun and honey time.
—Lucille Clifton, "new bones"

While Tayo learns that remembering is dangerous to the dominant culture because it is an act of resistance, for Sethe, Toni Morrison's main character in *Beloved*, memory is personally dangerous in multiple and complex ways. Among other things, *Beloved* connects historical rage, trauma, resistance, and the process of "rememory" for African American slaves and their descendants with hunger, starvation, feeding, and chronic overeating. The trauma of domestic and sexual violence on the female body becomes even more complicated by slavery and its aftermath. Specifically, Morrison's use of food and hunger imagery addresses the relation of the dysfunctional body to oppression and historical memory, an issue of importance to medicine. It is no coincidence that Velma Henry, in *The Salt Eaters*, experiences the apocalyptic vision of herself in Africa under the knife of female genital mutilation as she is coming through an important healing passage. Nor is it surprising that before Avey Johnson, in *Praisesong for the Widow*, reconnects with her history, she makes a painful and humiliating middle passage of her own, imagining herself as one of the slave bodies suffering with countless others in the "hot, airless dark." Or that Ciel Turner, in *The Women of Brewster Place*, at the height of her fever, is rocked by Mattie Michael, through time and memory to that place where mothers had dashed their babies' brains on the sides of slave ships to save them. Even Tayo sees the face of his ancestors in his so-called enemy and cannot pull the trigger (as he is having a so-called nervous breakdown). History extends itself through and in the body's memory. In *Beloved*, Sethe, the proud mother-slave, escapes and murders her "already crawling?" baby rather than allow the slave owner to recapture her, only to be haunted first by the ghost and then by its embodied form as a grown child. And Sethe's body bears the burden of that haunting in such a way that she nearly dies from it.

For Morrison, the social pathology undergirding the institution of slavery is inextricably linked to the physical, emotional, and spiritual pathologies of bodies that deny themselves food (as Sethe does in her obsession with feeding the ghost-child, Beloved) or chronically over-eat (as Beloved does in her desire to become "real") or simply live with an abiding and nameless hunger (as Denver, Sethe's surviving daughter, does). Marked in and on the bodies of slaves and their descendants, the institution of slavery itself is figured as an infecting agent of illness, much as abolitionist writing saw "slavery as a poison or disease that affects both the body politic and the body natural of each citizen."[1] Curiously, in *Beloved*, one of the manifestations of that illness is the relatively quotidian, quiet starving or excessive eating that today sends scores of women to treatment centers, therapy, and self-help groups and is typically considered a problem of middle-class white women.[2] In Morrison's hands, however, the issue is not control of food in order to create superior bodies, but the *survival* of bodies rendered inhuman and useful only for work and reproduction under the economy of slavery.

What does it mean that a novel set in the slave era employs representations of overeating, starvation, and complicated notions of embodiment? Unlike contemporary theories of women and eating disorders, which tend to focus on low self-esteem, childhood abuse, and other family dysfunction as etiological factors, and even those that place eating disorders within a social context, *Beloved* adds the dimension of historical memory and institutionalized, internal racism. I am not suggesting that Morrison is particularly interested in revising current notions of women and eating disorders in *Beloved*, but that her use of the imagery raises important questions about the nature of such disorders and their connection not just to the individual body (or the familial body) but to the body politic as well. Becky Thompson, in her book on women of color and eating, argues that "portraying [eating problems] as individual 'disorders' rather than as responses to physical and psychological distress is part of a historical tendency to mislabel the results of social injustices as individual pathologies."[3] Morrison creates both—a pathologized body and the reality of gross social injustice—refusing to separate the two.

In the 1980s, a body of work by women began looking at food, eating (or dieting), and the function of slenderness along with its relation to gender and social control.[4] In *Beloved*, however, Morrison appropriates overeating and starvation as tropes for the marking of historical memory on the bodies, minds, and souls of African Americans. The use of food imagery in *Beloved*, which is set in Ohio before the Civil War, is a synthesis of current concerns about the body's enslavement in eating disorders and the historical moment of the legal and literal enslavement of bodies. The returned ghost-child, murdered by her mother, fantasizes Sethe "chew[ing] and swallow[ing]" her, but conversely, "Beloved ate up [Sethe's] life, took it, swelled up with it, grew taller on it" (250).[5] Barbara Schapiro points out that "everywhere in the novel, the fantasy of annihilation is figured orally; the love hunger, the boundless greed, that so determines the life of the characters also threatens to destroy them."[6] As boundaries erode by way of food transactions, Morrison interrogates the limits of human interdependence and its extremes of symbiosis.

In addition, food in *Beloved* provides yet another frame for analysis of the destructive mechanism of internalized racism. Sethe's body itself becomes the site of racism's agency, turning against itself as she slowly starves, carrying out the brutal work of dehumanization rooted in slavery, but here unaided by slave owners or cruel overseers.

Instead, racism is maintained by and finds fulfillment in Sethe's body as she becomes literally consumed—enslaved—by Beloved's hunger. For Denver, the starvation is less literal, but the loss of boundaries and a sense of self, as well as her tremendous hunger for Beloved to recognize and bestow identity on her, is no less significant.

Surrounding the women's individual hungers are the sounds of "voices that ringed 124 like a noose" (183). These voices come from "the people of the broken necks, of fire-cooked blood and black girls who had lost their ribbons. . . . What a roaring" (181). The sounds of the "sixty million and more" play like a drone throughout the novel, never letting readers forget that the individual pain and horror represented in *Beloved* cannot possibly be comprehended without a historical and social context. While James Berger argues that historical trauma is "introduced into the narrative primarily through the figure of the returning and embodied ghost,"[7] it is also mapped on Sethe's body in the shape of the "tree" that was left on her back after the whip lashes had healed and in her slowly starving body after Beloved returned. The voices that ring the house—the potentially liberating memory of historical outrage and atrocity—become paradoxically the noose that makes possible the perpetration of more injustice and suffering, and it is replicated inside the house as the two women become so tied to Beloved and her rage that they are nearly destroyed.

Within the corrupt logic of slavery, Sethe—and all slaves—must be considered as non- or subhuman for the system to maintain itself. To justify commodification, slaves must be seen as *bodies* only. Susan Bordo observes that slavery deepens the already powerful dehumanization of racism, declaring that "the legacy of slavery has added an additional element to effacements of black women's humanity. For in slavery her body is not only treated as animal body but is *property*, to be 'taken' and used at will. Such a body is denied even the dignity accorded a wild animal; its status approaches that of mere matter, thing-hood."[8] Thompson describes "the existential nightmare of slavery," where "no self was legally recognized, and therefore the body could not exist for the self either."[9] In *Beloved*, Sethe and Denver repeat the existential nightmare as they become enslaved to Beloved's demands, and they cease to exist for/as/to themselves.

To complicate things, the slave body, maintained solely to work for a white master, historically carried within it the potential of becoming an anti-body under racism's yoke, one that could lose its ability to resist the infection of slavery and its dehumanizing commodification, ultimately turning against itself. Even though the female slave body was accorded value only as a commodity that added to the owner's capital, Sethe resisted, choosing and loving the man with whom she would have children (rather than being arbitrarily marked and used as a breeder). No small matter, this. As bell hooks observes, "The choice to love has always been a gesture of resistance for African Americans."[10] She asks, "What form could love take in such a context [as slavery], in a world where black folks never knew how long they might be together? Practicing love in the slave context could make one vulnerable to unbearable emotional pain."[11] Later Sethe escaped with those children when their survival was at stake. As a slave, she not only loved fiercely and courageously but had carried that courage into resisting "thing-hood," so much so that she fled Sweet Home plantation in her final month of pregnancy, her back ripped open by the whip. This rage to survive, however, later turns against her when that resistance leads her to be haunted by guilt for the murder. Killing her "already crawling?" baby and attempting to murder her other children to save them from slavery, Sethe becomes crushed by rage turned to guilt. Ironically, Sethe fulfills racism's function, much as an antibody would in an immune system—a system of resistance—when that system breaks down, leaving it open to serious, often fatal illness.

Baby Suggs, Sethe's gifted mother-in-law, knows that the slave body is ultimately disposable once its utility is gone. Moreover, a slave body that loves itself is subversive, dangerous to a society that relies on slave capital. For this reason Baby Suggs leads the community in a body-loving, body-affirming worship each week, telling her people that "the only grace they could have was the grace they could imagine" (89) and that imagination and self-love were acts of powerful resistance because they flew in the face of racist (and slaveholding) beliefs and practices.

> "And O my people they do not love your hands. Those
> they only use, tie, bind, chop off and leave empty. Love
> your hands! Love them. Raise them up and kiss them.
> Touch others with them, pat them together, stroke them on
> your face 'cause they don't love that either. *You* got to love
> it, *you*! And no, they ain't in love with your mouth. Yonder,
> out there, they will see it broken and break it again. What
> you say out of it they will not heed. What you scream from
> it they do not hear. What you put into it to nourish your
> body they will snatch away and give you leavins instead.
> No, they don't love your mouth. *You* got to love it." [88]

"They," the white world, will deny nourishment to the African American body, much as Beloved finally does to Sethe. In this powerful homily, Baby Suggs critiques at once slavery and racism, situating them in human evil, and invokes the slave body as human—created to be powerful, nourished, and beloved.

For Sethe, however, who has attempted to shut down the memories of slavery at Sweet Home and the killing, the "beloved" one is not her body but an Other, the insatiable ghost who comes to haunt and destroy her. Beloved quickly becomes the "they" who "do not love your flesh" but "despise it," as Baby Suggs says. Resistance in Baby Suggs's terms—self-love—dissolves as Sethe becomes more and more isolated from the community and fights to keep memory submerged, leaving her vulnerable to the ghost's demands. Beloved is a drug; with her, Sethe believes she has found the elixir of forgetting. Instead of self-love and a nurturing community, Sethe embraces Beloved as a tonic for the pain of slavery and for the lacerating memories of the murder. It is not the *heroism* of her past that haunts Sethe ("collected every bit of life she had made all the parts of her that were precious and fine and beautiful, and carried, pushed, dragged them through the veil, out, away, over there where no one could hurt them" [163]), but the guilt. This guilt is reinforced by the community's complicity in Sethe's isolation and by Paul D's condemnation when he later learns what had happened. Sethe's need to be exonerated allows Beloved to become a totalizing force in her life and thus to fulfill racism's agenda of annihilation of the strong Black woman-self Sethe had been in the past. Indeed, Sethe's attempt to satisfy Beloved becomes a form of self-consumption, as her own body begins to break down from lack of food (that Beloved compulsively eats instead).

Beloved's monstrousness is, in many ways, a projection of Sethe's own perception of herself as the monstrous mother as it is constructed in nineteenth-century racist discourse. The nineteenth-century ideal of domesticity and the effacing, nurturing (white, middle-class) mother throws into bold relief Sethe's actions, making them seem even more horrible. Sethe yearns and fights for her children's freedom, but within slavery and the discourse of her time, she is forced to see herself only as murderous. Mae Henderson says, however, that at the heart of Sethe's struggle is a desire for counter-narrative: "Sethe must compete with the dominant metaphors of the master('s) narrative—wildness, cannibalism, animality, destructiveness. In radical opposition to these constructions is Sethe's reconceptualized metaphor of self based on motherhood, motherliness, and motherlove."[12] As she works toward another way of seeing herself, Sethe struggles with the dismembered bits of her past in the images of the internalized narrative, and thus they are intolerably painful to her. The master narrative only allows her to see herself as that mother who murders and drives away her children. Thus, her heroism is eclipsed by her notion of herself as devouring mother—ironically reversed as the devoured child returns to devour her and her surviving daughter.

The triad of women—Sethe, Beloved, and Denver—enacts the power of racism to govern bodies through desire. Sethe permits her guilt to be embodied in Beloved and to turn itself against her. But Sethe is vulnerable for multiple reasons, not the least of which is her desire to heal her sundered motherhood, especially through feeding. In addition, she is separate from the community. Shunned by them because of what they perceive as her pridefulness, Sethe's isolation renders her almost without resources to resist the conflicts embodied in and reflected by the ghost. This governing power is enacted in Sethe's and Denver's almost total loss of identity and obsessive desire to keep Beloved present by feeding her overweening hunger. Bonnie Winsbro believes that Beloved's own lack of identity allows her to become a mirror for "the conflicted identity of the person who perceives her."

> Belief in the life of the human spirit after death sustains and consoles the ex-slaves living in and around 124 Bluestone by providing them with a sense of connectedness with those loved ones who have passed on. Such belief, however, when distorted by guilt, jealousy, or excessive love or need, can transform the spirit of a loved one from a benign presence into a vindictive, possessive, threatening, consuming monster—a projection, that is, of one's own internal conflicts.[13]

Beloved's presence, together with the women's desire for her, functions as the force to keep Sethe and Denver starving, without identity, without boundary—to keep them from full humanity. As Michel Foucault says of this kind of power, it is not necessarily about one person or persons holding a "consolidated and homogenous domination over others," but as

> something which circulates, or rather as something which only functions in the form of a chain. It is never localised here or there, never in anybody's hands, never appropriated as a commodity or piece of wealth. Power is employed and exercised through a net-like organisation. And not

only do individuals circulate between its threads; they are always in the position of simultaneously undergoing and exercising this power. . . . In other words, individuals are the vehicles of power, not its points of application.[14]

It is not that individuals never wield power or that power is never used by individuals to subjugate others, but that the mechanisms of power are far more complex than a reified notion of power might suggest. In addition, governing happens through desire, and it is through desire that power functions and is given agency. Sethe, Denver, and Beloved become the means of racism's diffuse and circulating power, as they become locked in a self-destructive and isolated loop, moving inexorably toward annihilation. And the point is that this self-destruction is not just about the mind, but about the body as well. Sethe's body, and to a lesser extent Denver's, becomes the site of racism's dirty work. In *Beloved*, eating, feeding, and starving all work as tropes to complicate the African American female body's relationship to history.

When Paul D comes back into Sethe's life years after they had been slaves at Sweet Home plantation, he observes that her eyes are "like two wells into which he had trouble gazing," and he remarks to himself that they "needed to be covered, lidded, marked with some sign to warn folks of what that emptiness held" (9). Sethe seeks to fill her emptiness after Beloved returns as a child by feeding her at all costs. She does this to satisfy her own need to obviate the trauma, to erase the memory of her slave past and to have not only the *memory* of Beloved's murder dissolved but also the very act itself, and to find a way back to that sense of herself as a (fiercely) loving mother. As long as Beloved remains embodied, Sethe is "excited to giddiness by the things she no longer [has] to remember" (183), since Beloved "understands it all. I can forget how Baby Suggs' heart collapsed; how we agreed it was consumption without a sign of it in the world. Her eyes when she brought my food [to prison], I can forget that, and how she told me that Howard and Buglar [her young sons who had since run away from home] were all right but wouldn't let go each other's hands" (183–84).

Not only is Sethe haunted by her notion of herself as a monstrous mother and trapped by the burden of slavery's history, but also, she later realizes, she is haunted by her past as a daughter. Much as a trauma survivor would do, Sethe suddenly remembers, while talking with Beloved, "something she had forgotten she knew." This was "something privately shameful that had seeped into a slit in her mind" (61): the time Nan, the woman who cared for her after her mother was hanged, told her that her mother had "thrown away" all of her children but Sethe; "the one from the crew she threw away on the island. The others from more whites she also threw away. Without names, she threw them. You she gave the name of the black man. She put her arms around him. The others she did not put her arms around. Never. Never. I am telling you, small girl Sethe" (62). For Sethe, this moment of memory is much like the Auschwitz survivor for whom her testimony, her remembering, marks a moment of profound change. Unlike the concentration camp survivor, however, for whom remembering is a "breaking out of Auschwitz even by her very talking," there is no breaking away for Sethe. Her newfound knowledge is "not simply a factual given that is reproduced and replicated by the testifier, but a genuine advent, an event in its own right";[15] but it leaves her still trapped in the frightening knowledge that her mother, too, murdered her children. The lone survivor of her brothers and sisters, Sethe struggles under the weight of that and other memories (significantly figured as food), which she futilely fights.

> She shook her head from side to side, resigned to her rebellious brain. Why was there nothing it refused? No misery, no regret, no hateful picture too rotten to accept? Like a greedy child it snatched up everything. Just once, could it say, No thank you? I just ate and I can't hold another bite? . . . But my greedy brain says, Oh thanks, I'd love

more—so I add more. And no sooner than I do, there is no
stopping. [70]

Beloved's advent is so powerful precisely because she has the power—
or so Sethe thinks—to alter the past and thus to change Sethe's sense
of self. Reversing the process of her hungry, greedy brain eating the
terrible memories, Sethe compulsively feeds Beloved instead, eventually at the expense of her own body. With Beloved's presence, Sethe
becomes fixed, not with resisting or rewriting the master narrative,
but appeasing it—as manifested in her frantic attempts to please
Beloved. Within the discourse of oppression, Sethe's memories cannot come together in a healing counternarrative but continue to
haunt her with the unspoken (and unspeakable) possibility that she
has always been the monstrous mother and is the daughter of a
monstrous mother as well.

Sethe's driving hunger to feed Beloved is also linked to the violent
and traumatic interdiction of maternal desire she experienced at
Sweet Home, what Lynda Koolish calls a "rupture of maternal love,"
when Schoolteacher's nephews held her down and "took [her] milk."
One obvious and powerful way of resisting thinghood, under the
terms of slavery, is to nurture one's own child. Koolish argues that
this rupture is

> signified not only in the murder of Beloved but also in
> Sethe's frantic, failed attempt to provide sufficient breast
> milk to her nursing babies. The extraordinary unquench-
> able thirst and hunger of Beloved is the mirror of Sethe's
> obsession with getting milk to her daughter, enough milk,
> milk she alone could provide. . . . Even before the theft of
> her breast milk . . . Sethe's breasts did not—could not con-
> tain milk enough to feed all who hungered.[16]

The need to feed one's child is so elemental that Sethe's desire becomes another way she is rendered vulnerable to Beloved's power to
overtake her. The theft of her milk and Sethe's response to it signals

the profoundly complicated relationship of maternal desire to the commodified female slave body. Paul D's incomprehension at the punishment Sethe received for telling on the boys is eclipsed by Sethe's outrage at the original act itself.

> "After I left you, those boys came in there and took my milk. That's what they came in there for. Held me down and took it. I told Mrs. Garner on em. . . . Them boys found out. . . . Schoolteacher made one open up my back, and when it closed it made a tree. It grows there still. . . ."
> "They used cowhide on you?"
> "And they took my milk."
> "They beat you and you was pregnant?"
> "And they took my milk!" [17]

The boys' act underscores Sethe's function as a slave: to produce food for whites even as they consume her. The maternal slave body becomes yet another function in the economy of slavery—providing a valuable resource to whites—motherhood stripped of agency, a motherhood of absence. Thus, in the terms of the master narrative, Sethe becomes the terrible mother doubly, not only because she kills her child, but also because she subverts the slave economy by doing so. This act of resistance complicates and intensifies Sethe's guilt in the eyes of the law: she is not only a monster of a mother, but she is also an enemy of the state.

It is no accident that Beloved "laps devotion like cream" (243) and that for Sethe, Beloved represents the opportunity to try to reclaim her desired role as nourisher and undo not only the murder but the theft of her milk. It is by way of the desire to nourish and nurture her children that racism's power overtakes Sethe through Beloved. As a slave woman, Sethe simply cannot win. As the mother who denies herself, she begins to approximate the prescribed role for nineteenth-century women, but it nearly kills her. Thus the novel exposes the catch-22 for Sethe. As long as she attempts to negotiate her identity as mother to Beloved within the crucible of nineteenth-century (white) domesticity and the institution of slavery, her sense of self is eroded more and more.

Arriving from under a bridge, literally just born from the water, Beloved walks into Sethe's and Denver's lives exhausted and violently thirsty. Concurrently, upon seeing Beloved in the yard, Sethe's bladder fills "to capacity" and bursts forth, much as it would if her water had broken from the womb. Significantly, Sethe's first observation is that Beloved is "poorly fed" (51). Indeed, Beloved's craving for the sweets ("sugar could always be counted on to please her" [55]) and other foods with which Denver and Sethe ply her suggests that those foods are only appetizers; what she truly wants is Sethe herself, as her eyes "lick," "taste," and "eat" Sethe (55). Beloved explains to the lovestruck Denver that Sethe is "the one. She is the one I need. You can go but she is the one I have to have" (76). As she attempts to feed Beloved (and thus quell the pain of memory), Sethe slowly starves. The first thrill of realizing that Beloved had "come back to her," and, ironically, her belief that she would never have to be haunted by the memories again, turns to anguish as Beloved becomes both accusing and increasingly demanding. "Beloved . . . said 'do it,' and Sethe complied. . . . Beloved accused her of leaving her behind. Of not being nice to her, not smiling at her." The present becomes conflated with the past as Sethe tries to explain her actions to Beloved, who only throws the history of slavery and hunger in her face:

> And Sethe cried, saying she never did, or meant to—that
> she had to get them out, away, and that she had the milk all
> the time and had the money too for the [grave] stone but
> not enough. That her plan was always that they would all
> be together on the other side, forever. Beloved wasn't inter-
> ested. She said when she cried there was no one. That dead
> men lay on top of her. That she had nothing to eat. [241]

Storytelling becomes another "way to feed" Beloved, and so Sethe becomes locked to her not only through food but by constantly keeping Beloved entertained. Sethe's connection to the ghost child becomes symbiotic as her need for forgetting and mercy grows in proportion to Beloved's rage to be re-membered, embodied and always fed. But while Sethe is desperate to "beat back the past," she also is "loaded with [it] and hungry for more" (70). The burden of the past haunts her as much as the disembodied baby ghost had and as Beloved now does. As hungry as she is to be a mother to Beloved, she is also desperate to make sense of the past, to "rememory" it, and in so doing, to loosen its hold on her. Beloved's demands on Sethe, however, become more and more intense, "and when Sethe ran out of things to give her, Beloved invented desire" (240). She wants Sethe's company; she dresses in Sethe's clothes, imitates her, and even carries herself "the same way down to the walk, the way Sethe moved her hands, sighed through her nose, held her head," and sometimes, for Denver, "it was difficult . . . to tell who was who" (241). But Beloved grows in size, becoming obese, and Sethe shrinks. Sethe cannot sleep and loses all interest in taking care of her physical body, sitting in a chair, "licking her lips like a chastised child while Beloved [eats] up her life, [takes] it, [swells] up with it, [grows] taller on it" (250). And so Sethe diminishes with the force of her own hunger. Rather than consuming food, Sethe *becomes* food for the embodied ghost. Thus, when Sethe coughs up something that is not food but is a part of her own body, her daughter Denver finally realizes that she is literally dying of starvation.

When Beloved comes to live at 124 Bluestone, Denver herself becomes a ghost of sorts. Having known loneliness for most of her life, she is absolutely starved for community. The house had become an island of isolation after the baby's murder, "no visitors of any sort and certainly no friends" for twelve years (9). Baby Suggs's withdrawal and eventual death severed Denver's connection with life-affirming energy. Her loneliness is figured in the text also as hunger. Her secret hideaway is an "emerald closet" made up of the space within "five boxwood bushes ringed round . . . closed off from the hurt of the hurt world, [where] Denver's imagination produced its own hunger and its own food, which she badly needed because loneliness wore her out. *Wore her out*" (29; emphasis in original). Denver describes her extreme loneliness and the undercurrent of fear that she lived with always, and how she only had the disembodied ghost for company all her growing up years.

> I love my mother but I know she killed one of her own
> daughters, and tender as she is with me, I'm scared of her
> because of it. . . . And there sure is something in her that
> makes it all right to kill her own. All the time, I'm afraid
> the thing that happened that made it all right for my
> mother to kill my sister could happen again. I don't know
> what it is, I don't know who it is, but maybe there is some-
> thing else terrible enough to make her do it again. I need to
> know what that thing might be, but I don't want to. What-
> ever it is, it comes from outside this house, outside the
> yard, and it can come right on in the yard if it wants to. So
> I never leave this house and I watch over the yard, so it
> can't happen again and my mother won't have to kill me
> too. [205]

But "whatever it is" *does* come back and, through the mechanism of desire and fear, is nurtured, held, and maintained in both Sethe's and Denver's lives. Beloved is she whom both Denver and Sethe assume they want when in fact she brings slavery's institutional energy: racism. Beloved's appearance sharpens Denver's sense of loneliness, and she becomes possessively attentive to the girl who arrives with a fever, "breathing like a steam engine" (53). In addition, Beloved defuses Denver's fear; for if Beloved was killed and has returned, then Denver can maintain the illusion that she is (relatively) safe from the thing that made Sethe kill once before. Accordingly, Denver's atten-tiveness becomes an obsession with Beloved as she nurses her back to health, and Denver forgets to eat or even to visit her former hideaway, the emerald closet.

Intensely erotic, Denver's gaze at Beloved becomes "food enough to last. But to be looked at in turn was beyond appetite; it was breaking through her own skin to a place where hunger hadn't been discovered" (118). Denver also "nurs[es] Beloved's interest like a lover whose pleasure was to overfeed the loved" (78). In such passionate moments, Denver loses all sense of herself; her "skin dissolve[s] under that gaze," and she "float[s] near but outside her own body" (118). And yet, while she imagines herself disembodied, she also has the sense of being seen, made visible by Beloved ("You are my face. You are me" [216]). Denver's enslavement to Beloved is manifested in the lengths to which she would go to preserve the loss-of-self/reconstruction-of-self that Beloved catalyzes.

> The present alone interested Denver, but she was careful to appear uninquisitive about the things she was dying to ask Beloved, for if she pressed too hard, she might lose the penny that the held-out palm wanted, and lose, therefore, the place beyond appetite. It was better to feast, to have permission to be the looker, because the old hunger—the before-Beloved hunger that drove her into the boxwood and cologne for just a taste of a life, to feel it bumpy and not flat—was out of the question. Looking kept it at bay. [119–20]

For Denver, "anything is better than the original hunger" that grew out of the ordeal of witnessing her own and her brothers' near-extinction at their mother's hands and Sethe slitting Beloved's throat. Loneliness and the isolation that came when Sethe refused the community's sympathy ("trying to do it all alone with her nose in the air" [254]) motivated Denver's retreat with her mother into their domestic world. Denver's panic at the thought of losing Beloved, whom she imagines to be her only tie to a textured life, is ironically rooted in her own loss of self.

> If she stumbles, she is not aware of it because she does not know where her body stops, which part of her is an arm, a foot or a knee. . . . "Don't," she is saying between tough

swallows. "Don't. Don't go back." . . . Now she is crying because she has no self. Death is a skipped meal compared to this. She can feel her thickness thinning, dissolving into nothing. She grabs the hair at her temples to get enough to uproot and halt the melting for a while. [123]

It is, however, Beloved's ephemeral body that cannot exist without the bodies of them. Yet both Denver and Sethe believe that without Beloved they will in some way cease to exist. All three characters struggle to be real, articulated human beings, but they look for that realness to come from the other. Beloved's realness is contingent on Sethe's and Denver's isolation and unfed hungers—always connected to the institution (slavery) and events (atrocities at Sweet Home) that led up to her murder in the shed. For Sethe, realness depends on Beloved exonerating her for the murder, something she is incapable of doing, since she embodies not only her own rage but the rage of millions of dead slaves. In attempting to find freedom in Beloved, Sethe entraps herself in a life-draining enterprise, for it is from a cipher that she attempts to feed her hunger for forgiveness. For Denver, the realness she seeks exists in relationship; only the relationship is with a ghost who drains the very sense of identity necessary to maintaining human connections. She pleads with Beloved, "You are my face; I am you. Why did you leave me who am you?" (216).

By mapping the hungers of all three characters, we can also see the lineaments of resistance and healing. Sethe and Denver, while marked by the history of slavery, are also survivors. But institutional barbarity moves in and through bodies, its symptoms manifesting in various ways. In *Beloved*, the trope of hunger and overeating foregrounds how the body simultaneously adapts to and resists oppression. As Sethe and Beloved grow more tightly entwined and their boundaries dissolve, hunger (both Beloved's and Sethe's) and food render Sethe virtually invisible to herself. Sethe seeks to ease her guilt and grief, to become the mother/self she could not be under slavery, by surrendering her volition to Beloved. Similarly and paradoxically, as Denver feeds Beloved in order to experience herself, she loses all sense of herself except as she is reflected in Beloved.

Sethe's insistence on feeding her own children, on guarding her "milk," has isolated her more and more from the community. This isolation is compounded by the community's own judgment of the murder and their isolation of Sethe for what they perceive as her prideful ways, creating the chasm in which Beloved thrives. I think Koolish is correct when she asserts that the community is protecting themselves from the terrible knowledge of "what Sethe's act implicitly reveals"—that the consequences of slavery were many times worse than Beloved's murder—and it is for this reason that they reject Sethe.[17] I am reminded of Nancy Scheper-Hughes's description of a woman in jail for murdering her infant son and one-year-old daughter in Brazil: "The infant had been smothered, and the little girl hacked with a machete. . . . Face to face with the withdrawn and timid slip of a girl (she seemed barely a teenager), I made myself bold enough to ask the obvious: 'Why did you do it?' She replied as she must have for the hundredth time, 'To stop them from crying for milk.'"[18] What the women in Sethe's community did not want to face was slavery's corollary to the *delíro* in the Brazilian Bom Jesus community that drove the young woman to kill her children simply to save them from such pain.

While Sethe's and Denver's hungers are a different kind of *delíro*, it is not surprising that food also becomes a means to community and healing and inverts the existing structure of isolation at 124 Bluestone. Feeding Beloved only makes her more monstrous, but when Denver and Sethe accept the gift of food from women in the community, they necessarily open their hands, a gesture signifying the end of the hold Beloved needs to stay embodied. Once they let go of her, Beloved floats away. They cannot do this alone, though, and it is only through a process that begins when Denver observes Sethe and realizes the seriousness of the situation: "The flesh on her mother's forefinger and thumb was thin as china silk and there wasn't a piece of clothing that didn't sag on her. Beloved held her head up with the palms of her hands, slept wherever she happened to be, and whined for sweets although she was getting bigger, plumper by the day. Everything was gone except two laying hens." Driven by the greater fear that they would all starve to death, Denver "step[s] off the edge of [this] world" (239) into another that awaits her, drawing upon the affirming spirit (a different kind of ghost-presence) of her grandmother Baby Suggs, who has come to help her make the frightening crossing from isolation into community.

> "But you said there was no defense."
> "There ain't."
> "Then what do I do?"
> "Know it, and go on out the yard. Go on." [248]

There is no defense against racism and death, and Baby Suggs knows this well; but she also knows the absolute necessity of being for and with one another, feeding and being fed, being a healing community in the face of evil.

After Denver walks out of the house, she goes to her former teacher. When Lady Jones provides rice, eggs, and tea, she becomes the first to break the community's silence. For one as hungry and isolated as Denver has been, the act of receiving food from another woman represents the beginning of a radically disruptive new way of thinking: "having a self to look out for and preserve" (252). In this moment, Denver begins to create a new discourse for herself, one that resists the master narrative within which the body could not exist for the self. As food begins to appear in the yard regularly, Denver leaves home to return the empty baskets to each woman, and she is welcomed back into the community with every visit. Each woman leaves a sign of her identity on her gift of food so that Denver will not only return thanks and the empty bowl or pan but will have direct contact, thereby reestablishing her links to the world beyond the isolation of 124 Bluestone. The names inscribed on the baskets and bowls of food proclaim identity, selfhood, and bodies who want to keep themselves, along with Denver and Sethe, alive.

Denver is not the only one who breaks through to another narrative, however. The women begin a process of healing memory as they piece together stories of life with Baby Suggs, "the days when 124 was a way station, the place they assembled to catch news, taste oxtail soup, leave their children, cut out a skirt" (249), and they soften in their condemnation of the perceived pride that filled Sethe's house. As they remember the ways they had come together for support and sustenance at 124 Bluestone earlier, they experience themselves coming together to provide it this time. They learn from Janey Wagon (with whom Denver has begun working as a domestic) just why Sethe is in such straits: "Sethe's dead daughter, the one whose throat she cut, had come back to fix her" (255). In addition, by facing and drawing courage from their own memories of violation and trauma, the women build solidarity with Sethe and find within themselves empathy for her suffering that creates a bridge over and out of the endlessly circulating guilt and self-destructive power that Beloved's presence maintains.

Through fear for her mother, Denver has slowly allowed herself to be nourished by others. Her compulsion to cling to Beloved's presence is every bit as painful and difficult to break as an addiction, but she cannot and does not have to struggle with this in a vacuum. First Baby Suggs's spirit and then strong African American women intervene to empower Denver. It is in the act of moving out of isolation and allowing herself to be nurtured and fed by other women that Denver's healing begins and that the chain binding Sethe and Denver to Beloved is weakened.

Beloved complicates the notion of community, however. One could reasonably argue that Denver, Beloved, and Sethe form their own community. Obviously, just because it is "community" does not make it liberating. Theirs is closed, tightly constructed, and ultimately destructive. The text bids readers ask, What are the terms of a healthy community? In the closed community, boundaries blur and are transgressed as identities break down. As Denver leaves this community for another, she goes where she is fed, moving from starvation to being nurtured by hands other than her own. But Denver has to take the first step. She draws on the affirming spirit of Baby Suggs and moves out into the dangerous but potentially healing world. In addition, the women outside have done their own shifting, seeing Sethe's plight differently from before. Without them, Sethe is still locked in Beloved's hold.

As they gather in her yard and Sethe hears the sounds of the women (all thirty of them), which connects them to the rage of the sixty million dead slaves, she responds and comes to the door. The power expressed by the women is similar to that which led Sethe to kill her daughter rather than consign her to a life of slavery; unfocused and isolated, however, it turned against her and led her to forget what the women's voices awaken in her.

> They grouped, murmuring and whispering, but did not step foot in the yard. Denver waved. A few waved back but came no closer. Denver sat back down wondering what was going on. A woman dropped to her knees. Half of the others did likewise. . . . Among those not on their knees, who stood holding 124 in a fixed glare, was Ella, trying to see through the wall, behind the door, to what was really in there. . . . Ella had been beaten every way but down. She remembered the bottom teeth she had lost to the brake and the scars from the bell were thick as rope around her waist. She had delivered, but would not nurse, a hairy white thing, fathered by the "lowest yet." It lived five days never making a sound. The idea of that pup coming back to whip her too set her jaw working and then Ella hollered. [258–59]

Ella's yell cracks the shell of silence around 124. While Denver is the link between the community and Sethe, Ella first connects directly with Sethe through the hell of her own experience, and the other twenty-nine women quickly join her.

Although she had previously shunned Sethe, Ella taps into her own knowledge of suffering and leads the rest of the women into a powerfully articulated anger. "Instantly the kneelers and the standers joined her. They stopped praying and took a step back to the beginning. In the beginning there were no words. In the beginning was the sound, and they all knew what that sound sounded like" (259). The healing fury of the community is set against the evil of racism, not the bodies on and in which racism has done its evil. As Ella remembers—with power—her rape and the birth of the "hairy white thing" and her resistance to becoming a victim, she focuses that same rage and resistance against the rapaciousness of Beloved. She also connects her own acts of infanticide with Sethe's and sees them as both profoundly painful acts of resistance to dehumanization and the master narrative that structures such dehumanization. This fury is not leveled against the dead child but against the monster racism has created and that Sethe's desire has permitted, the monster that seeks to devour her and Denver.

Collectively, the women drive Beloved from 124, thus ending the murderous, nooselike isolation that has choked Sethe and Denver. An agent in her own healing, Sethe finally walks out of the house and into the group of women; they do not drag or even escort her out. She allows herself to be re-membered into the community but not dissolved into it. This process is figured as a reverse of Beloved's coming, when Sethe lost her water and became lost in Beloved. Here the sound of the women's voices "[breaks] over Sethe and she tremble[s] like the baptized in its wash" (261). Her figural rebirth back into a community of strong women protects Sethe when she mistakes Mr. Bodwin (the man who "had kept [her] from the gallows in the first place") for the slave catcher from years before. As she runs toward him with an ice pick, reenacting what had happened so long ago, the women "make a hill. A hill of black people, falling," and prevent her from killing him (262).

And so Sethe's obsessive, isolated feeding of Beloved ceases with the departure of the embodied ghost. She has eaten food made and offered by women from the community, has allowed herself to be fed, and has been strengthened enough to receive the gift of their inter-vention when the women come into her yard to "save her from a futile cohabitation with loss."[19] In this way, Sethe has opened her hands to receive food and to let Beloved go when the women come to drive her away. The erased self is reinscribed by food and the wom-en's presence. Food allows Sethe not only to survive physically, but it becomes the means for her to re-join a powerful community, rich in historical memory and knowledge. As Sethe and Denver leave their isolation, they also experience what Beloved had taken from them: a sense of identity as well as personal boundaries. They both have the opportunity to discover and re-learn interdependence within this community as Denver's first acceptance of food begins to weaken racism's power that bound the women to the dangerous and embod-ied ghost.

Sethe's grief at losing Beloved is intense; but Paul D tells her it is not Beloved, but Sethe herself, who is her own "best thing." This is not a concept to be internalized easily. Yet Sethe begins to reclaim her identity and her memories, and the annihilating work of racism is interdicted through her own and the community's powers of re-sistance. Beloved's memory remains, but it is a *rememory*, one that has the potential to cure rather than destroy. For Beloved's power as embodied suffering—of the sixty million and more—cannot and should not be forgotten. Once Sethe no longer needs to run from the memories, however, she can use them as she creates a life-affirming resistance to racism, based on presence rather than loss. It is in human bodies that the evil of racism plays itself out, and it is through the process of becoming re-membered (into oneself and into a healing community) and allowing the self to be nurtured—fed—that the body encounters the power to resist destruction. In *Beloved*, food and feeding have the potential both to destroy and to heal. Morrison's text becomes a space in which history's horrible record of racism and slavery is played out within female bodies and through hunger. Be-loved the child will never be forgotten, should never be forgotten, just as the "sixty million and more" should not be forgotten. But neither should their memory continue slavery's bitter legacy. The women have brought food. The noose is loosened. Sethe the starved becomes Sethe the fed. And she is on her way, quite possibly, to becoming Sethe her own best thing.

Medicine makes no appearance in this novel, and yet it is an important text for medicine in considering the role of history and ongoing oppression on sick bodies. Imagine a medical team trying to diagnose Sethe or someone like her, or simply trying to feed her or medicate her depression (brought on by guilt? by murder? by having been a slave? an ancestor of a slave?). Simply understanding the complexities of Sethe's state of mind, the ghost notwithstanding, would be a formidable task. *Beloved* insists that along with the social and cultural context, the legacy of historical trauma must not be forgotten. At Cook County Jail, where I regularly teach creative writing workshops, I see hundreds of women who bear the scars of a collective history—not unlike Sethe's scars. They may not have literal or embodied ghosts in their lives, but many are nonetheless haunted. When the medication cart comes wheeling down the hall and the women line up to be dosed, I wonder not only what brilliance, what resistance, or what rage is being temporarily put to sleep, but what ghosts as well. It is impossible to imagine a world of health where memory is asleep or absent. Facing memory is hard work, and *Beloved* illuminates the many ways that this work is made even more complex when the memory involves trauma, marginalization, and historical oppression. Help for Sethe comes from a community of women who can relate to her injuries—both the whip scars on her back and the network of scars that so constricts her heart. While women like Sethe might not end up in sophisticated private practices, they are likely to show up in clinics, emergency departments, and certainly jails and prisons. Rhodessa Jones discusses a well-known fact: that incarcerated people (overwhelmingly from the lowest socioeconomic social sectors) are held in jails and prisons with little or no real attempts at healing:

I think people delude themselves. They think that if they
slap an adult on their hands, hold them somewhere for six
to twelve months, they're not going to come back to jail.
Given their crimes and the reasons that they're there: poverty, sickness, all that stems from pain and loss and lack of
self-esteem—they think they're not going to come back?
And in the course of time, nobody—their captors, the
gatekeepers, the keyholders—gets them to tell their story.[20]

It is important that medicine understands, at the very least, the
importance of story, of community, and it must help patients, when
possible, find the appropriate means to this. Morrison's novel, however, like the others in this study, reminds readers that without social
change, healing is difficult, mostly impossible. I know wonderful
clinicians and other health care workers at Cook County Hospital
who have added their voices to various arenas of social struggle,
seeing themselves as both health care workers and advocates for a
different world. But it should not just be Cook County clinicians and
others like them on urban front lines who raise their voices for social
change. They and other members of the medical community must be
joined with (and supported by) women and men from the nonmedical community and work together to provide a social context within
which health at least has a possibility to flourish.

Saving You the Doctor's Way Would Kill You

Seeing and the Racial Body in Louise Erdrich's *Tracks*
and Toni Morrison's *The Bluest Eye*

4

> I saw through the eyes of the world outside of us. I would not speak our language.
> —Louise Erdrich, *Tracks*

> "What about your eyes?"
> "I want them blue."
> —Toni Morrison, *The Bluest Eye*

As Sethe is haunted—literally—by the legacy of slavery and finds healing in a return to a community of memory, characters in Louise Erdrich's *Tracks* and Toni Morrison's *The Bluest Eye* are made ill by racism and poverty but never find their way to a healing community. In addition, the novels are, in large part, about seeing, examining the effect of a kind of seeing that is refracted through the lens of racism by the subjects of racism themselves. Erdrich's Pauline Puyat and Morrison's Pecola Breedlove are made crazy from their dealings with racism and suffer from an internalized self-hatred that is upheld and maintained by racist social and cultural structures within which they live, especially those institutions designed to be helping agents. One such institution is medicine. In both novels, the brief appearance of physicians suggests their function as agents of racism. In their ignorance of it, the doctors perpetuate racism and "help" becomes dangerous to the characters. Significantly, the strongest characters in these novels maintain their health at a safe remove from institutionalized medicine. In *Tracks* and *The Bluest Eye*, unlike Silko's Tayo, Pauline and Pecola do not experience healing but instead become progressively more off center; they become embodiments of a world sickness, one of whose symptoms is racism. As all of the issues dealt with in this study, these are not simply historical realities from a distant past, nor are they dystopian fantasies; but they have their roots in very real and present social concerns. For example, the *American Journal of Orthopsychiatry* devoted a special section of its January 2000 issue to a discussion of racism and mental health. Numerous studies have documented the impact of racism on self-esteem and the deleterious effect on psychological well-being.[1] Others have pointed out how institutional racism affects minority groups through mental health policy and practice.[2]

Both Erdrich and Morrison ground the destruction of their characters' bodies and minds in the harsh realities of race, class, and gender oppression. They illuminate in story what Paul Farmer calls "the mechanisms through which large-scale social forces crystalize into the sharp, hard surfaces of individual suffering."[3] It is clearly not Native American or African American life that is pathologized, but the dominant society in which characters must struggle to survive. Both writers are clear about where the illness lies, and they create characters and scenes that provide contrapuntal readings to the stories of despair that are embodied in Pauline Puyat and Pecola Breedlove. In providing alternative stories, the texts throw the consequences of internalized racism into bold relief. In Morrison's and Erdrich's hands, racism is the root of illness that has as one of its symptoms the desire to destroy or erase the body. Erdrich's Pauline and Morrison's Pecola function as critiques of a model of assimilation that demands of its subjects an erasure of identity. In fact, Pauline and Pecola are figured as the site of racism's genocidal extremes, and they themselves become agents of what seeks to undo them: racism, complicated by poverty and gender-role bias.

In a climate of such hostility, Pauline and Pecola learn to see themselves through the eyes of their oppressors as flawed or even inhuman and consequently aspire to be like their white oppressors. Both novels suggest that Pauline and Pecola suffer illnesses that are, as Silko says of Tayo's in *Ceremony*, "part of something larger" than individual or family pathology. Pauline Puyat, seeing herself through the eyes of whites, attempts to escape her heritage and, in the process, adopts an extreme, self-mutilating Christian asceticism. Similarly, Pecola Breedlove's deep belief in her ugliness leads her to the conclusion that the only means to salvation (for the "sin" of not being white) is the acquisition of blue eyes, a gesture that requires the imagined obliteration of her body (and, of course, her mind). Both characters go crazy with the burden of seeing and of not seeing themselves. Their way of seeing, and its concomitant self-hatred and self-erasure, is maintained and reproduced by dominant social systems in which they are situated.

Set in the early twentieth century, *Tracks* creates a chronicle of the Anishinabe community from 1912 to 1924 in North Dakota. Part of an interlocking series of novels including *Love Medicine* (1984), *The Beet Queen* (1986), and *The Bingo Palace* (1994), *Tracks* is the third and most historical of the tetralogy. It traces the struggle of the Anishinabe to survive and continue their hold on tradition in the face of shifting U.S. policies toward Native Americans. *Tracks*, says Nancy Peterson, is a novel that "enables readers to think through the issues and the stakes involved in the crisis of history surrounding Native Americans."[4] The larger story of survival through hard freezes, deadly influenza, smallpox, tuberculosis, near-starvation, and land swindles provides the context for the narrative of Nanapush's family, including the powerful Fleur Pillager. Pauline's increasing alienation and destructiveness, however, drives a great deal of the novel's action.

The Bluest Eye, set in Lorain, Ohio, during the early 1940s, chronicles the life of the Breedlove family through the perspectives of two African American girls, Claudia McTeer and her sister Frida. The novel focuses especially on Pecola, "a black girl who wants blue eyes as a symbol of beauty and therefore of goodness and happiness."[5] All of the characters in the novel confront in different ways (and with varying degrees of success) the privileging of whiteness and Euro-American concepts of beauty. The narrator, Claudia McTeer, becomes insightfully aware of the consequences of loving whiteness more than the self, but Pecola and her mother never escape the pull of dominant white images of romance and beauty, particularly those constructed cinematically. Like *Tracks*, *The Bluest Eye* is a novel about vision, and Morrison explains its problematic aspects: "The interest in vision, in seeing, is a fact of black life. As slaves and ex-slaves, black people were manageable and findable, as no other slave society would be, because they were black. So there is an enormous impact from the simple division of color—more than sex, age, or anything else. The complaint is not being seen for what one is."[6]

Norman Yetman observes that the assimilation model has provided the "dominant conceptual framework in the analysis of American ethnic and racial relations."[7] This model assumes that the racial/ ethnic minority will be absorbed into the dominant group without consequence and with full privilege accorded to any member of the U.S. citizenry. Yetman cites Milton Gordon's continuum of assimilation, however, that describes the model's extremes: genocide/ extermination (less autonomy) and separatism (more autonomy). Between the extremes lie exclusion/expulsion, caste, transmuting pot, melting pot, and pluralism. Yetman reminds readers that "a policy of genocide was one of several pursued by dominant whites in their effort to wrest control of the country's vast lands from the Indians," and that by the turn of the twentieth century, the United States had reduced the Indian population to near-extinction.[8] (Yetman does not, however, mention the role of disease in this program of extermination.) Although it is not as drastic as institutionalized genocide, Yetman points to slavery as an example of a nonetheless damaging node on the assimilation continuum; it is the caste system that "accepts the existence of minorities . . . but subjugates them and seeks to confine them to inferior social positions."[9] What Yetman alludes to but does not elaborate on is the instability of these positions. Certain historical moments and perceived exigencies dictate differing responses to assimilation(s). Our current paranoia about terrorism is a good example. Where Muslims, especially those of Arab descent, were more or less tolerated, after September 11, 2001, they were moved to the much more dangerous node of exclusion/ expulsion in the United States.

In both *Tracks* and *The Bluest Eye*, genocide as well as exclusion and expulsion are manifest in the textual representation of racism and—for Pauline and Pecola—its consequent mental disequilibrium. Mental distress, however, in these instances becomes written on the body: in both texts the characters not only become more and more mentally disturbed but their bodies also become inscribed with racism's destructive agenda. Self-hatred becomes self-mutilation. The characters themselves carry out racism's function as they turn away from their own bodies (and their communities). Throughout *Tracks*, the imagery of frozen, sick, dying, and mutilated bodies—and their historical context—serves as a background for Pauline's own self-mutilation. Cinematic imagery and the idolatry of the white, blonde, blue-eyed female body in *The Bluest Eye* situates Pecola's mental illness in its cultural and social context.[10] Racist society scarcely needs weapons other than the psychological tools of this kind of seeing that demands allegiance to white Euro-American standards of beauty and power.

Neither Pauline nor Pecola comes into contact with institutionalized medicine, but medicine is present in both novels through the experiences of other characters and provides a lens through which to interpret Pauline's and Pecola's illnesses. Both novels implicitly challenge individualistic explanations often relied on by Western medicine as reasons for mental illness, and they root etiology in the racist and oppressive history of which each character bears the scars, rather than in their individual circumstances. For these writers, individual histories and contexts are inseparable from greater political and social sickness. The authors carry out the agenda that Howard Waitzkin has challenged medicine to follow: make explicit the connection between "personal troubles" and social problems.[11] In Erdrich's and Morrison's hands, mental illness becomes yet another symptom of a society that is itself an infecting agent. Just as the body cannot be separated from the mind and the mental illness marks itself on each character's body, neither can the illness be separated from the world, the society in which those characters live. Pauline and Pecola become racism's bodies, performing the annihilating functions of racism—on themselves and, in *Tracks*, on the community. Where the novels discussed in Chapters 1, 2, and 3 set forth a record of resistance to medical and other colonization, *Tracks* and *The Bluest Eye* demonstrate the consequences of not resisting.

Tracks is told in the counterpointing voices of Nanapush, a tribal elder and healer, and Pauline Puyat. Significantly, Nanapush's narrative is addressed to his granddaughter, Lulu, and begins with "we." Pauline's narrative is addressed to no one but herself and indicates her isolation and alienation from the community. In Pauline, Erdrich creates a voice through which to examine the politics of assimilation, "a voice that echoes hegemonic history."[12] Pauline, like Tayo, is of mixed-blood heritage and never quite fits into the communities she inhabits. Her family, the Puyats, were "skinners in the clan for which the name was lost" (*Tracks*, 14).[13] To get attention, Pauline relies on "telling odd tales that created damage" (*Tracks*, 39). Sounding a little like Tayo's beloved cousin, Rocky, Pauline declares, "I wanted to be like my mother, who showed her half-white. I wanted to be like my grandmother, pure Canadian. That was because even as a child I saw that to hang back was to perish. I saw through the eyes of the world outside of us. I would not speak our language" (*Tracks*, 14).

Pauline lives in what bell hooks calls "a state of forgetfulness, embracing a colonized mind so [she] can better assimilate into the white world."[14] Pauline, however, is not simply in a passive state of forgetfulness. She actively works to erase all sense of her native heritage, "a victim of accelerated acculturation": "Her loss of cultural and personal identity becomes apparent in her frenzied attempts to identify with white European ideals, and her growing religious fanaticism emerges as a response to an alienated reality."[15] Pauline does not see that she is in need of healing. Rather, she conflates guilt over what she considers her past sins with a more far-reaching guilt that hinges simply on the "original sin" of not being white.

Pauline moves to Argus to live with her Aunt Regina, her cousin Russell, and Regina's common-law husband, Dutch James. Although her father "scorned [her] when she would not bead [and] refused to prick [her] fingers with quills, [when she] hid rather than rub brains on the stiff skins of animals," Pauline declares that she "was made for better" (*Tracks*, 14). She insists on learning the more dignified tradition of lace making from the nuns in Argus but ends up sweeping floors in a butcher shop and taking care of Russell instead.

Tracks traces the roots of Pauline's increasing isolation and, while foregrounding racism, also examines the role of other events in Pauline's life. For example, Pauline's fascination for the unassimilated Fleur Pillager turns to horror and then guilt when she witnesses Fleur's poker partners violently raping her in retaliation for her consistent wins. In this act, Fleur's body becomes the site on which the text of racial destruction is written as she cries out "in the old language," resisting violence through the words of her forebears. Pauline and Russell hear Fleur's cries, her "hoarse breath, so loud it filled [her]," and their names "repeated over and over among the words" (*Tracks*, 26). Later, Pauline remembers the scene and guiltily believes that she was Fleur's "moving shadow . . . the shadow that could have saved her" (*Tracks*, 22).

A tornado, believed to have been sent by Fleur as revenge, occurs the next night. As Pauline and Russell run for shelter, they realize that the men have locked them out of the safe haven of the meat locker.

> Russell howled. They must have heard him, even above the driving wind, because the two of us could hear, from inside, the barking of that dog [inside the locker]. . . . It was Russell, I am sure, who first put his arms on the bar, thick iron that was made to slide along the wall and fall across the hasp and lock. He strained and shoved, too slight to move it into place, but he did not look to me for help. Sometimes, thinking back, I see my arms lift, my hands grasp, see myself dropping the beam into the metal grip. At other times, that moment is erased. [*Tracks*, 27]

The children survive, and all but one of the men die in the freezer. Fifteen-year-old Pauline will keep the secret of her and Russell's rage and punishment of the men's violence and neglect. She will also internalize and suffer from the guilt of what she perceives as her role in the rape and the men's murder.

The rape and its aftermath signify more than drunken revenge for Fleur's winnings, however. The men cannot stand Fleur's strength or her independence. Moreover, the rape is a symbolic act of violence against indigenous ways. But in Fleur's mouth, the "old language" pours forth as the men batter and rape her, and she will not be silenced. Fleur's utterances, her resistance to the rape of her language, liberate Russell and Pauline momentarily from the moorings of complicity in domination, and they consequently lock the men in the freezer. But Pauline's ensuing guilt signals her divided sense of loyalty, as well as a sense of diminishing agency. Although Pauline refuses to speak anything but English, Fleur's cries in the native tongue become, for her, the repressed that returns to haunt her in nightmares and visions.

Pauline finds a vocation to work with the dying of her community. She convinces the widow Bernadette Morrisey ("the one who washed and laid out our dead" [*Tracks*, 54]) and her brother Napolean to take her on as a helper. She begins to sit on deathwatch with Bernadette, and her nightmares intensify. With the nightmares, troubling religious and erotic stirrings begin to emerge.

> I relived the whole thing over and over. . . . Every night
> when my arms lowered the beam, it was my will that bore
> the weight, let it drop into place—not Russell's and not
> Fleur's. For that reason, at the Judgment, it would be my
> soul sacrificed, my poor body turned on the devil's wheel.
> And yet, despite that future, I was condemned to suffer in
> this life also. Every night I was witness when the men
> slapped Fleur's mouth, beat her, entered and rode her. I felt
> all. [*Tracks*, 66]

Pauline's incipient religious masochism has roots in a racist agenda: the sacrifice of her body and soul. Indeed, Pauline's lurid images set the stage for her attachment to death. Not until Pauline witnesses

Mary Pepewas's dying do the awful dreams finally cease. She is fascinated by the process and her perceived power over it: "I saw very clearly that she wanted to be gone. . . . That is why I put my fingers in the air between us, and I cut where the rope was frayed down to string" (*Tracks*, 68). Pauline is ecstatic as Mary dies, and she spends the night in a tree, emerging with the conviction that she had "the merciful scavenger's heart" and was "a girl of bent tin," one who "made death welcome" (*Tracks*, 69, 71, 69). Susan Pérez Castillo argues that Pauline represents "death as the only space of refuge for her people,"[16] a point in keeping with the trajectory of her self-annihilating tendencies that begin to occur after the rape.

As Pauline's sexuality begins to emerge, she finds herself jealous of Fleur and her husband, Eli, whose passionate sex life together is well known in the community. Herself a bundle of sexual ambivalence and confusion, Pauline works a "spell" on Eli and Bernadette's teenage daughter, Sophie, compelling them to have prolonged, ecstatic sex one afternoon as Pauline watches, "pitiless," imagining that she is controlling them as though "they were mechanical things, toys, dolls wound past their limits" (*Tracks*, 84). Later, when Pauline realizes that Sophie's father plans revenge on Eli, she fears that she has gone too far. This slight rupture in Pauline's destructiveness signals a flicker of something important remaining in her: a kind of resistance that allows her to counter her projected self-hatred. Pauline quickly retreats into her fear of bringing trouble to herself and stays quiet, however, and the momentarily self-protective gesture is lost altogether by the end of the novel.

Pauline's repressed sexuality is figured in the "miraculous" tears of the Virgin Mary (tears only Pauline sees) that she scoops up. These tears are frozen from being outside, much as Pauline's sexuality is frozen, and resemble "ordinary pebbles of frozen quartz." Brooding for a long time over the cause of the tears, Pauline comes to believe that it was because the Virgin had known "the curse of men": "In God's spiritual embrace She experienced a loss more ruthless than we can imagine. She wept, pinned full-weight to the earth, known in the brain and known in the flesh and planted like dirt. She did not want

Him." Pauline herself had begun having sexual relations with Napolean (Bernadette's brother) and was terrified to find that she "could not resist more than a night without his body" (*Tracks*, 95).

Internalized racism and self-hatred write themselves on Pauline's body when she becomes pregnant and tries to abort. She is stopped only by Bernadette, who promises to keep the baby after he or she is born. Naming the unborn child Marie (for the Virgin), Pauline experiences her pregnant body with pure hatred and despair, and she attempts to strangle the emerging baby with her legs during the delivery. She nearly succeeds in killing the baby until Bernadette ties her to the bed and uses two large spoons to drag Marie to her first breath. Pauline never touches the baby and leaves Bernadette's house, as soon as she is able, for the convent on a hill above the reservation. In attempting to kill Marie, Pauline almost succeeds in serving the cause of genocide, destruction of the racialized body.[17]

In the convent, Pauline embraces and is rewarded for her sadomasochistic asceticism. With Pauline, "mortification of the flesh" becomes the theological justification she needs. Many ascetics such as the Desert Fathers, St. John of the Cross, and St. Teresa of Avila, for example, "viewed pain and suffering—both physical and mental—as a prerequisite or concomitant condition to the *unio mystica*,"[18] validating Pauline's (at first) slightly offbeat and, later, self-destructive practices. It is striking how much of Pauline's narrative resembles that of the Desert Fathers: "Every affliction tests our will, showing whether it is inclined to good or evil. . . . If you do not want evil thoughts to be active within you, accept humiliation of soul and affliction of the flesh; and this not just on particular occasions, but always, everywhere and in all things."[19] St. Teresa of Avila reports in her spiritual writings that at one time she was "tormented for five hours with such terrible interior and exterior pains and disturbance that it didn't seem to me I could suffer them any longer."[20] David Morris notes that the visionary pain of Catherine (of Siena), Teresa (of Avila), and Sebastian becomes "a means of knowledge, offering access to an otherwise inaccessible understanding."[21] For Pauline, however, this particular spiritual epistemology is distorted and comes in the form of visitations by a racist Jesus: "He said that I was not whom I had supposed. I was an orphan and my parents had died in grace, and also, despite my deceptive features, I was not one speck of Indian but wholly white. He Himself had dark hair although His eyes were blue as bottleglass, so I believed" (*Tracks*, 137). Jesus' blue eyes serve as a reproach to Pauline for her brown ones, and it is no wonder that she is desperate to learn from him that her Native American family is not really hers. Individuals and institutions (even and especially the Church) have done nothing to help Pauline question her love of blue eyes and white skin.

Erdrich inserts a tale into the narrative that mimes Pauline's own self-destruction and its roots, anatomizing internal racism and calling into question institutional complicity. Nanapush tells Pauline of a time when he had guided a buffalo expedition for whites, and the animals had "misunderstood" what was happening. The surviving buffalo "lost their minds," turning against one another in their fear: "They bucked, screamed and stamped, tossed the carcasses and grazed on flesh. They tried their best to cripple one another, to fall or die. They tried suicide . . . [and] to do away with their young" (*Tracks*, 140). Imagining that she has seen the same thing on the reservation, Pauline believes that she has been called by a white Jesus to save them from their "Indianness." But as Hertha Wong points out, "Pauline's madness is to recognize her female Chippewa self as Other, even as she tries to destroy it."[22]

The imagery of sick and dying bodies weaves through both Pauline's and Nanapush's narratives. The colonizers bring smallpox and influenza, weakening the Indians so that what the severe winters have not killed, the diseases will. Pauline's madness has its roots in a system that a priori dismisses the value of people of color—and at its extreme demands annihilation. For example, when Lulu, Nanapush's granddaughter, walks in the snow with thin shoes and suffers severe frostbite on her feet, the physician ("another something [Nanapush] did not want" [*Tracks*, 167]) insists on amputation. Unhappy at having been called by the priest to an Indian family, the doctor becomes furious at Nanapush's resistance to what would amount to immobilizing Lulu. "No quiet child, no pensive thing who could survive without running. You were a butterfly, a flash of wit and fire, a blur of movement who could not keep still. Saving you the doctor's way would kill you" (*Tracks*, 168). Recalling Eric Cassell's insistence that when physicians attempt to impose a treatment without knowing the patient's life context, they often inflict rather than alleviate suffering, this physician not only does not have the vaguest idea of who Lulu is, but it never occurs to him to think of her as a complex human being.[23] He grudgingly offers amputation (mutilation) and commands Fr. Damen to "reason with the idiot" (*Tracks*, 168) when Nanapush refuses. Instead, Nanapush takes on the job of facilitating Lulu's healing himself, banishing the doctor and spending days bathing her feet in water and pickling salt, using purifying smoke, and telling her stories through the long and painful nights until she can walk again. Not only is Nanapush an alternative healer who can see the consequences of the doctor's unthinking treatment, but the healing gesture is also an act of profound and loving resistance in this instance. Nanapush knows that the doctor's role in racism is so deeply ingrained in him that to ignore, eliminate, or mutilate the bodies of Indians seems normal. Lulu's lifeworld is as invisible to this doctor as Tayo's was to the doctors in the Veterans Hospital.[24]

Nanapush's power of resistance and identification with his culture and history are far removed from Pauline's experience. Where Pauline has a gift of sight in her work with dying people, her way of seeing herself and her world is fractured and self-destructive. It is also destructive to the community. Pauline imagines that Fleur Pillager's power makes her a special target of God. Her fascination with Fleur coupled with this conviction leads Pauline to harass her frequently. When Fleur goes into labor prematurely, Pauline is present but fails to help. Rather than refuse outright, however, Pauline begins to shake as Fleur cries for help; Pauline becomes clumsy and "forgets" what the healing alder plant Fleur calls for looks like. After scalding her own leg with boiling water, she concludes that "the Lord overtook [her] limbs and made them clumsy. . . . It must have been His terrible will" (*Tracks*, 157). Fleur loses the baby and almost dies as Pauline unhelpfully passes out and hallucinates traveling through time and space with Fleur. Pauline awakens to find herself pinned to the floor by a knife between her legs thrown by a weak but outraged Fleur in a figural reenactment of Fleur's earlier rape by the drunken men.

Soon after this incident, Pauline's self-destructiveness reaches new heights: "Shattering ice from the buckets in the kitchen, I scraped my hand raw. But I continued to smash my fist into the water until the water told the story" (*Tracks*, 164). Months later, Pauline interrupts a healing ceremony for Fleur's depression (in the aftermath of the baby's death). Claiming that she had been sent to "prove Christ's ways," she plunges her hands into a ceremonial pot of boiling water and herbs: "She lowered them farther, and kept them there. Her eyes rolled back into her skull and the skin around her cheeks stretched so tight and thin it nearly split. If she opened her mouth . . . pure steam might blast into the air. Moments passed. Then she shrieked, jumped. She clawed straight through the flimsy tent walls, scattering the willow poles, collapsing the blankets and skins around us all" (*Tracks*, 190). An act of self- and community hate is "faith" in Pauline's mind, and the chaos left at the healing site becomes the figure for Pauline's mark on the community and the community's inability to reach her.

Indeed the greater damage is to Pauline herself. Christ comes to her one night dressed as a peddler, "with a pack on his back full of forks, scissors, and paper packets of sharp needles" that he "tried . . . out upon [her] flesh" (*Tracks*, 193). Pauline finally becomes the embodiment of self-loathing, one who is nothing without pain. Seeing herself through white eyes, refusing to speak her own native language, Pauline is encompassed by pain. It is no wonder that she is "hollow unless pain filled [her], empty but for pain" (*Tracks*, 192), an emblem of racism's disabling and annihilating work.

Pauline's Jesus has blue eyes, and Pecola Breedlove worships them in whites. Morrison's story, like Erdrich's, constructs a text of racism's annihilation as well as a narrative counter to that text. *The Bluest Eye* traces the etiology of the Breedloves' pain, rooted in racism and poverty. As Eliott Butler-Evans says, "The novel is primarily concerned with the issue of cultural domination" as it follows "the disintegration of Pecola's life."[25] But it is also a story of resistance and the conditions in which resistance can grow and be maintained, as well as the conditions that stifle it.

While Pecola's disintegration has roots in poverty and racism, it is specifically linked to racist representations of beauty and romantic love, supporting both white society's and the Breedloves' belief in their ugliness. Self-hatred spills over onto hatred of those who resemble the self, as happens with Pecola's mother, Pauline.

> The Breedloves did not live in a storefront because they were having temporary difficulty adjusting to cutbacks at the plant. They lived there because they were poor and black, and they stayed there because they believed they were ugly. . . . The master had said, "You are ugly people." They had looked about themselves and saw nothing to contradict the statement; saw, in fact, support for it leaning at them from every billboard, every movie, every glance.
> [*Eye*, 34]

The sense of ugliness is figured as illness when the narrator describes the home as an infectious place where the family "fester[ed] together" (*Eye*, 31). Even inanimate objects such as furniture could provoke physical illness in such a home, and the effects of poverty on the poor are likened to the body in pain:

> An increase of acid irritation in the upper intestinal tract, a light flush of perspiration at the back of the neck as circumstances surrounding the piece of furniture were recalled. The sofa, for example. It had been purchased new, but the fabric had split straight across the back by the time it was delivered. The store would not take responsibility. . . . Like a sore tooth that is not content to throb in isolation, but must diffuse its own pain to other parts of

the body—making breathing difficult, vision limited,
nerves unsettled, so a hated piece of furniture produces a
fretful malaise that asserts itself throughout the house and
limits the delight of things not related to it. [*Eye*, 32–33]

The narrative shifts from a focus on the family's pain to the social
pathology that is the infecting agent. Poverty and racism function as a
pestilence, infecting, isolating, and shading the Breedloves' world
with distress.

Elaine Scarry's description of the body in pain applies to the body
under racism's own form of torture. "Regardless of the setting in
which he [*sic*] suffers (home, hospital or torture room), and regardless
of the cause of his suffering . . . the person in great pain experiences his own body as the agent of his agony. The ceaseless, self-
announcing signal of the body in pain at once so empty and un-
differentiated and so full of blaring adversity, contains not only the
feeling 'my body hurts' but the feeling 'my body hurts me.' "[26] That
racism inflicts pain is no news. The way it inflicts pain—the sense of
self-hatred, self-alienation, and self-betrayal to which Scarry points—
indicates an unsettling similarity between racism and torture. The
Breedloves connect the visceral pain of poverty's conditions to their
own sense of personal anguish and thus believe what the dominant
culture already believes, that they are ugly to the core. Like the
terrified buffaloes that turn against one another in Nanapush's story,
Cholly and Pauline take out their fury and frustration on each other
and their children, becoming at the same time both wounded survivors and agents of torture.

Small wonder, then, that Pecola becomes obsessed with the "blue-
and-white Shirley Temple cup" when she lives temporarily with the
McTeer family. For Pecola, the only escape from the agony she has
known is flight to whiteness. Just as Morrison gives food significance
beyond sustenance in *Beloved*, she also does this in *The Bluest Eye*. In
attempting to internalize all that Shirley Temple represents, Pecola
furtively drinks an entire three quarts of milk from the cup to the
uncomprehending fury of Mrs. McTeer. Neither is it a surprise that

Pecola's mother (whom she calls "Mrs. Breedlove") identifies with white cinematic representations of beauty, romantic love, and success. Before Pecola's birth, she had used the movies as a way to ease her loneliness after moving from rural Kentucky to urban Ohio:[27]

> There in the dark her memory was refreshed, and she succumbed to her earlier dreams. Along with the idea of romantic love, she was introduced to another— physical beauty. Probably the most destructive ideas in the history of human thought. Both originated in envy, thrived in insecurity, and ended in disillusion. In equating physical beauty with virtue, she stripped her mind, bound it, and collected self-contempt by the heap. [*Eye*, 97]

When Pauline was five months pregnant with Pecola, she lost a tooth in the movie theater and viewed herself with disgust, "trying to look like Jean Harlow, and a front tooth gone." She marks her decline from this point: "Look like I just didn't care no more after that" (*Eye*, 98).

In the hospital ("so I could be easeful"), giving birth to Pecola, Pauline's encounter with physicians momentarily interrupts her unthinking self-contempt when they insult her by commenting that she and the other black women deliver their babies without pain, "just like horses" (*Eye*, 99).[28] Worse than invisible to the doctors on rounds, she refuses to confirm their racist assumptions, creating a text counter to the doctors' narrative: "I moaned something awful. The pains wasn't as bad as I let on, but I had to let them people know having a baby was more than a bowel movement. I hurt just like those white women. Just 'cause I wasn't hooping and hollering before didn't mean I wasn't feeling pain" (*Eye*, 99). This brief interjection of institutional medicine into the story's multiple narratives, much like the insertion of the white doctor in *Tracks*, implicates medicine's potential for the kind of erasure that, even though Pauline and Nanapush resist it, puts medicine at the service of racist agendas.

Another moment of resistance occurs in the novel when Claudia McTeer becomes ill and her overworked mother roughly, perhaps resentfully, cares for her. "No one speaks to me or asks how I feel," Claudia complains to herself. When her mother returns with Vicks salve, Claudia feels "rigid with pain" as a "hot flannel is wrapped about [her] neck and chest" (*Eye*, 13). When she vomits on the bedclothes and is chastised by her mother, Claudia cries, not realizing that her mother "is not angry at me, but at my sickness." Looking back on the incident, Claudia remembers the important, life-affirming image of hands in the middle of the night, "somebody with hands who *does not want me to die*" (*Eye*, 14; emphasis mine). This is the knowledge that supports Claudia's ability to interrogate the terms of Shirley Temple's cuteness and to reject her "because she danced with Bojangles, who was *my* friend, *my* uncle, *my* daddy and who ought to have been soft-shoeing it and chuckling with me" (*Eye*, 19; emphasis in original). This is precisely the kind of knowledge Pecola does not have. Claudia's revulsion at the blue-eyed baby dolls she receives for Christmas prompts her to dismember them, "to see what it was that all the world said was lovable" (*Eye*, 20). Pecola's dismantling impulses exist in stark contrast to Claudia's; Claudia destroys white dolls to understand what it means to be black rather than wishing to take herself apart piece by piece because she *is* black. Claudia also carries this impulse into her relations with white girls, and she is curious, but not worshipful, about "the magic they weaved on others. What made people look at them and say, 'Awwww,' but not for me?" (*Eye*, 22).

Rather than making Claudia's powerful critical move, however, Pecola, who has never experienced "hands that did not want her to die," worships whiteness. Instead of taking white dolls apart, Pecola symbolically attempts to internalize them and become them, much as she has done with milk in the Shirley Temple cup. Pecola also consumes Mary Jane candies as a way of escaping her black body and for a moment imagines herself ingesting the attributes of the little white girl on the candy wrapper. She fantasizes the "resistant sweetness that breaks open at last to deliver peanut butter—the oil and salt which complement the sweet pull of caramel. A peal of anticipation unsettles her stomach" (*Eye*, 41). Erotic in their power over her, the candies also—and more powerfully—appeal to her need to be someone she is not, to annihilate herself:

> Each pale yellow wrapper has a picture on it. A picture of little Mary Jane, for whom the candy is named. Smiling white face. Blonde hair in gentle disarray, blue eyes looking at her out of a world of clean comfort. The eyes are petulant, mischievous. To Pecola, they are simply pretty. She eats the candy, and its sweetness is good. To eat the candy is somehow to eat the eyes, eat Mary Jane. Love Mary Jane. Be Mary Jane. [*Eye*, 43]

Pecola learns over and over that she is not and never will be Mary Jane. For example, entering the kitchen of the household where her mother works, Pecola sees her mother fawning over the white child (who calls her Polly). When she accidentally spills the hot berry cobbler her mother has just made for her charge, Pecola is violently driven from the house by her enraged mother:

> Most of the juice splashed on Pecola's legs, and the burn must have been painful, for she cried out and began hopping about just as Mrs. Breedlove entered with a tightly packed laundry bag. In one gallop she was on Pecola, and with the back of her hand knocked her to the floor. Pecola slid in the pie juice, one leg folding under her. Mrs. Breedlove yanked her up by the arm, slapped her again, and in a voice thin with anger abused Pecola directly. . . . Her words were hotter and darker than the smoking berries. [*Eye*, 86–87]

Pecola is tortured, multiply burned, and humiliated, deepening her shame and self-hatred. The "smoking berries" function as a smoking gun of guilt, pointing at Pecola for being nonwhite, poor, and simply not as beautiful as the soft little white girl in her freshly pressed nightgown. Morrison, however, ties Pecola's abuse to Pauline's own history: "The perversion of Pauline's nurturing impulses—her will-ingness to sacrifice her child for the sake of another woman's baby—is a direct consequence of her economic deprivation and of the rac-ism which lies at its root."[29]

Similar to Pauline Puyat in her turn to religious asceticism and self-inflicted torture, Pecola fantasizes about dismantling her body. When her parents fight violently, Pecola prays to disappear: "Little parts of her body faded away. . . . Her fingers went, one by one; then her arms. . . . Only her tight, tight eyes were left. They were always left." In attempting to bring peace to the house, Pecola has prayed to be "pretty," to have blue eyes, but to escape the hell of life at home, Pecola imagines annihilating herself.

> Long hours she sat looking in the mirror, trying to discover the secret of the ugliness, the ugliness that made her ig-nored or despised at school, by teachers and classmates alike. . . . It had occurred to Pecola some time ago that if her eyes . . . were different, that is to say, beautiful, she her-self would be different. . . . If she looked different, beauti-ful, maybe Cholly would be different, and Mrs. Breedlove too. Maybe they'd say, "Why, look at pretty-eyed Pecola. We mustn't do bad things in front of those pretty eyes."
> [*Eye*, 39–40]

Pecola's year of prayer for blue eyes culminates in her being raped and impregnated by her father and suffering her mother's violent retaliation.

Pecola turns to Soaphead Church, a self-proclaimed preacher, de-scribed as a "misanthrope" who "dallied" with the priesthood in the Anglican Church, who hated human contact but loved little girls' breasts. Promoting himself as "Reader, Adviser, and Interpreter of Dreams" (*Eye*, 130), Soaphead becomes a substitute for institu-tions of care within the community—church, family, school, and medicine—all of which have utterly failed Pecola. Unable to attend school because of her pregnancy, Pecola asks Soaphead to help her by making her eyes blue, and he feels "a surge of love and understanding" as well as anger that he is so powerless to help her, this "little black girl who wanted to rise up out of the pit of her blackness and see the world with blue eyes" (*Eye*, 137). Soaphead is wrong, however; Pecola does not want to see the world with blue eyes, but to be seen by them. As long as he persists in seeing her caught in "the pit of her blackness," he is, indeed, powerless to help her and culpable in her suffering. His solution is a bogus miracle in which Pecola witnesses a dog's excruciating death by poison, after Soaphead assures her that "if the animal behaves strangely, your wish will be granted" (*Eye*, 138).

Finally driven completely over the edge, Pecola gives birth to a baby that dies shortly afterward. "Lucky to be alive herself," say the townspeople, "the way her mama beat her" (*Eye*, 148), Pecola's brutalization is complete, but not before she nearly annihilates her own powers of seeing with her now "blue" eyes: "Look. I can look right at the sun. . . . I don't even have to blink" (*Eye*, 151). "The damage done was total. She spent her days, her tendril, sap-green days, walking up and down, up and down, her head jerking to the beat of a drummer so distant only she could hear. Elbows bent, hands on shoulders, she flailed her arms like a bird in an eternal grotesquely futile effort to fly" (*Eye*, 158). In a grotesque revision of the African folktale of the people who fly away from their enslavement back to Africa, Morrison creates a character broken and without hope, forever grounded.

Both Pecola Breedlove and Pauline Puyat see themselves and the world through the eyes of the dominant white culture, which at best renders them invisible and, at its worst, wants them dead. As they become more adept at seeing themselves through this lens, their self-annihilating tendencies become more pronounced. For both characters, their narratives—and their lifeworlds—become more and more fragmented until they are incoherent.

What, however, does this have to do with medicine? In not seeing how internalized racism works, medicine is doomed to reproduce it.

In *Tracks*, the doctor cannot consider an alternative to amputation; in *The Bluest Eye*, doctors cannot see that Pecola's mother is more than a foaling mare. Of course, not just race, gender, or ethnicity is at stake here, but the complication of class as well. Paul Farmer's work in Haiti has led him to observe, "The suffering of individuals whose lives and struggles recall our own tends to move us; the suffering of those who are distanced, whether by geography, gender, 'race,' or culture, is sometimes less affecting." Farmer adds that "to explain suffering, one must embed individual biography in the larger matrix of culture, history, and political economy."[30] Morrison and Erdrich construct stories by which readers may move closer to recognizing the complexity and intensity of such suffering as Pauline and Pecola experience and, in so doing, perhaps begin to close the distance between easily recognized experiences of suffering and the less recognizable suffering of an "Other." Otherness is, of course, an always shifting and unstable category based on a complex of interlocking factors, always calling on the difficult work of using Adrienne Rich's "lens of empathy." Both Pauline and Pecola are not unlike patients who might wind up in emergency rooms or psychiatric units. These two characters and their stories raise perhaps some of the most unsettling questions in this study, for neither of them has a foreseeable positive outcome. While Pauline at least has the convent (nutty as it is), Pecola is last seen by a compassionate but distant narrator who observes her staring open-eyed at the sun. Where is the healing community for Pecola? Where would be the resources to which medicine could turn if Pecola or Pauline were to appear at its door?

The suffering of Pauline and Pecola manifests itself in physical destruction and self-mutilation. What is important and disturbing about *Tracks* and *The Bluest Eye* is that the beliefs that both Pauline and Pecola hold—that white is superior, that to be of color is to be ugly and inferior—are so aligned with dominant beliefs that they are invisible and mostly uncontested. These internalized beliefs undergird Pauline's and Pecola's illnesses and might be missed—or worse, seen and ignored or even intensified—in a strictly biomedical analysis of etiology and treatment. C. R. Ridley, D. W. Chih, and R. J.

Olivera suggest using a cultural schema in the mental health profession to reduce unintentional racism, but this assumes that clinicians understand their own cultural biases and worldviews.[31] One study advises including the legacy of slavery and the history of racism in the United States as a way of better understanding the current health care issues of the African American population.[32] These suggestions and critiques indicate the need to go far beyond traditional psychiatric and psychological models in biomedical training and practice. But racism is not the only factor; otherness is at stake, and class differentials as well as race, ethnicity, sexual orientation, gender, and disabilities all may get in the way of seeing and hearing an Other. Without understanding the complicated issues someone like Pecola or Pauline brings to a medical encounter, a helping professional cannot draw on what resources do exist within the community. Furthermore, it is impossible to challenge the kinds of beliefs held by characters like Pauline and Pecola (*I am ugly, I need to be white, should be white, need blue eyes, need a different heritage*).

For both Pauline and Pecola, internalized racism is complicated because not only have they learned self-hate, but they also lack the resources to question it. It is the pernicious trait of racism that it not only supports the racialized Other in hating the self, but it also disallows a questioning of that self-hatred. In such a system, resistance *is* health, a kind of resistance that permits one to live intentionally against the grain of racism (dismantling racist structures rather than the self). Both Pauline's and Pecola's histories have misshaped their ways of seeing and disabled resistance. Pauline, believing that she must atone for the sin of not being white, obeys the message of racism, placing her faith in a white, blue-eyed Jesus who directs her to mutilate herself and to work mischief (and death) in her community. For Pecola, who also believes she deserves her misfortune because she is "ugly" and black, her failure to resist means that she internalizes racism, and her family's abuse of her only compounds that internalization. The extent to which medicine—and the community— leaves such skewed vision unexamined and unchallenged is the extent to which we are together complicit.

It Tried to Take My Tongue

Domestic Violence, Healing, and Voice in Sandra Cisneros's
"Woman Hollering Creek," Bebe Moore Campbell's
Your Blues Ain't Like Mine, and Sapphire's *Push*

5

> I saw disease.
> It closed doors, turned on light.
> It owned water and land.
> It believed in its country
> and followed orders.
> It went to work.
> It tried to take my tongue.
> But these words,
> these words are proof
> there is healing.
> —Linda Hogan, "Sickness"

> but she means to have what she
> has earned,
> sweet sighs, safe houses,
> hands she can trust.
> —Lucille Clifton, "to my friend, jerina"

In the novels discussed in the preceding chapters, characters in each text grapple with a variety of injuries or illnesses caused by deplorable social conditions: domestic and sexual violence, literal or figural enslavement, poverty, and the damaging socially constructed stories of who they are. Healing for them includes a process of refinding, retelling, and/or resisting dominant narratives based on race, ethnicity, gender, and class. In Sandra Cisneros's story "Woman Hollering Creek," Bebe Moore Campbell's *Your Blues Ain't Like Mine* and Sapphire's *Push*, each character discovers an alternative way of thinking about herself and her realities and a new language for telling her story. This new or newly rising language, along with her connection to a healing community, becomes part of the means of each character breaking away from the entrapment of domestic violence and sexual abuse.

While some of the silence around domestic violence has been shattered, current statistics suggest that not everyone is talking. The Department of Justice reports that more than 50 percent of women surveyed in 2000 had been physically assaulted. Intimate partners primarily perpetrate violence against women. Indeed, 64 percent of the women surveyed by the Department of Justice reported being raped, physically assaulted, and/or stalked by an intimate partner.[1] The World Health Organization states that one in five of the world's female population has been physically or sexually abused by a man or men at some time in her life.[2] Carole Warshaw insists that "for most women, the greatest risk of physical, emotional, and sexual violation will be from a man they have known and trusted, often an intimate partner."[3] In her groundbreaking study of domestic violence and trauma, Judith Herman connects the trauma of rape and domestic violence to that of war and torture. Commonalities exist, she says, "between rape survivors and combat veterans, between battered women and political prisoners, between the survivors of vast concentration camps created by tyrants who rule nations and the survivors of small, hidden concentration camps created by tyrants who rule their homes."[4]

Studies indicate that between 22 and 35 percent of women seeking care in hospital emergency rooms are battered. Further, 25 percent of women who attempt suicide or use an emergency psychiatric service have been battered, along with some 50 percent of women psychiatric outpatients and 64 percent of women psychiatric inpatients.[5] Warshaw writes that domestic violence is frequently ignored in emergency department settings even when it is obvious and "even in hospitals with established domestic violence protocols."[6] Instead, victims of battering are treated symptomatically and, in the case of ongoing episodes, are likely to be labeled pejoratively as a "crock" or "hysteric" or, at best, as someone with a "self-defeating personality disorder."[7]

Much as Warshaw critiques the medical discourse of domestic

violence, Kathleen J. Ferraro assesses the prevailing feminist discourse around the issue. Instead of focusing on the notion of personality disorder, Ferraro argues, the discourse frequently reproduces hierarchies based on race/ethnicity, class, and gender.

> In the United States, at the end of the millennium, "domestic violence" is a code for physical and emotional brutality within intimate relationships, usually heterosexual. As a code, it glosses the intricate, layered connections of power relationships built on race, class, and gender hierarchies, each tied in unique fashion to requirements of female dependency. These power hierarchies recede as the discursive focus abstracts acts of violence as a pathology to be remedied, separate from a critique of the relationships of dominance through which it is constituted. . . . Like other aspects of early second wave feminism, domestic violence discourse has been oriented toward the construction of a unified image of "battered woman" and "batterer."[8]

Ferraro goes on to insist that "feminist liberatory discourse has been overshadowed by a crime control discourse" that "undermines critiques of dominance through its focus on individual men."[9]

In another analysis, Renee Heberle draws on the work of Elaine Scarry to caution feminists about the political cost of bringing the "rape culture" into the public sphere. In her examination of the mechanisms of state power and the routine use of torture to create an image and fantasy of power, Scarry describes how torture is "useful to the regime beyond being a punishment for resistance."[10] Likewise, sexual violence against women is a "necessary tool deployed in the name of stabilizing the otherwise fragile edifice of masculinist power—creating its fictions but also enabling its material effects in the world."[11] Heberle worries that discourse about sexual violence reifies male dominance and shores up an illegitimate power, and she asks instead, "What if sexual violence were argued to signify the limits of patriarchy, rather than to represent its totalizing authority or power over women as a system?"[12] It seems to me, then, that in particularizing violence in the lives of female characters, revealing its interconnectedness to other forms and categories of oppression, *and* in constructing characters that resist and unmask male power, many novelists go far in subverting politically problematic discourse around domestic and sexual violence.

It is within this context that I have read "Woman Hollering Creek," *Your Blues Ain't Like Mine,* and *Push.*[13] In all three texts, a female character with few economic and educational resources experiences domestic and sexual violence. One character is Latina, one is white, and one is African American. All are poor. It is important to point out, however, that domestic violence is a system of control that cuts across racial, ethnic, class, and sexual orientation lines, affecting every community and category of women.[14] Although Herman points out that "when the victim is already devalued (a woman, a child), she may find the most traumatic events of her life take place outside the realm of socially validated reality[, and] . . . . her experience becomes unspeakable,"[15] she does, however, not take into account factors such as race, ethnicity and class, which compound and complicate such unspeakability. As Paul Farmer argues when discussing suffering, marginalized populations "are not only more likely to suffer, they are also more likely to have their suffering silenced."[16] It is the finding, or rediscovery, of voice, the emergence from silence, that interests me. What are the conditions that make this possible? What does such an emergence look or sound like? How is the emergence of voice a sign of healing or perhaps a healing phenomenon? And why should this be of interest to medicine?

Elaine Scarry, looking at the nature of extreme physical pain, describes what happens to language when intense pain, especially torture, is inflicted. The sufferer moves from language to incoherent utterances—moans, cries, and screams. It is, she argues, an experience where language is "unmade," a process where the body's pain becomes the entire world of the sufferer: "It is . . . intense pain that destroys a person's self and world. . . . [It] is also language-destroying: as the content of one's world disintegrates, so the content of one's language disintegrates; as the self disintegrates, so that which would express and project the self is robbed of its source and its subject."[17] Scarry also argues that the return of language becomes a world-making event, in which creativity, sentience, and agency are reborn. "To witness the moment when pain causes a reversion to the pre-language of cries and groans is to witness the destruction of language; but conversely, to be present when a person moves up out of that pre-language and projects the facts of sentience into speech is almost to have been permitted to be present at the birth of language itself."[18]

Although domestic violence is not usually categorized as torture, I agree with Herman that it should be (and I am aware of the problematics of saying so). Much of the dynamic is the same, even if the pain is not always as systematic or calculated as state-sponsored torture.[19] Silence is frequently the result of domestic and sexual violence, a silence that could be likened to the dismantling of language that occurs in torture. While the critiques of domestic violence discourse are politically important, much of the writing about healing and domestic violence focuses on silence and the search for voice, the emergence of a new language.

Ann Russo writes about her struggle to come to terms with the "multiple experiences of abuse throughout [her] childhood" and the importance of recognizing that survival and healing are integrally connected to the preexisting narratives about who we are, from where we came, and what is possible for us even to think. "Our experiences are shaped by the socially constructed stories that we tell about our lives. The stories are different depending on who we are—our experiences, our social positionalities, our historical and political contexts, and the available social narratives, as well as from whose perspective the stories are told."[20] In the instance of abuse, those narratives need to expand in order to frame what happened, she argues. Shame and guilt become transformed into something else when the language of resistance and struggle replaces them with a word like "rape," for example. Russo calls for politicized language that provides a larger analysis of what has happened and can provide tools for examining social institutions that collude and reproduce oppression. With new, politicized language, stories of pain, guilt, and shame can become narratives of resistance and even stories of abundance and possibility.

In "Woman Hollering Creek," *Your Blues Ain't Like Mine*, and *Push*, the characters move from relative silence to a resisting and empowered voice, or the beginnings of it, and only one does so within a medical context. In all of the texts, the growing ability to use language as a naming, defining tool becomes a primary healing agent, central to each character's emergence from powerless unspeakability to an empowered voice and consequent sense of personal agency. None of the characters makes this healing move alone. All of them first encounter another woman or women and begin the emergence from silence within a community where they may share common pain and together find the language that will heal and empower them. In each text, however, the characters' acquisition of such empowering language falls along a spectrum. In "Woman Hollering Creek," Cleófilas finally and simply asks for help and in so doing turns the tears of La Llorona into laughter. Lily Cox, in *Your Blues Ain't Like Mine*, learns, with the help of her daughter, to resist her battering husband. Only gradually does she replace the language of collusion and her husband's lies with her own truth. Finally, Precious Jones, of *Push*, offers perhaps the clearest example of the power of language and naming to disrupt and transform the experience of the nearly unspeakable pain she has endured all of her life.

In a story that reverses the dream of immigration to the United States and constructs it as a domestic nightmare, Sandra Cisneros also creates an alternative to the traditional story of La Llorona. In it, Cleófilas moves from her home in Mexico to live with her husband across the border in Seguín, Texas, *el otro lado* (the other side).[21] Belonging to a demographic group of women particularly vulnerable to domestic violence, Cleófilas speaks no English and, once she is married, is allowed no contact with her family of origin.[22] As an immigrant woman isolated from her family, she has even less access to information, services, and legal protection than nonimmigrant women have. Cleófilas's isolation becomes its own form of abuse when extended family and friends become complicit as they move farther away from her or deny that her realities are anything but the norm. While Cisneros, in her earlier collection *The House on Mango Street*, tells stories of characters who are silenced or constricted as a result of gender oppression and, in some cases, domestic violence, Jacqueline Doyle notes that Cleófilas's story "extends and revises such histories, opening a borderland space where old myths take on new resonance and new forms and where new stories are possible."[23]

Cleófilas learns quickly that the love she had imagined is nothing like that which the movies and *telenovelas* had promised. In Mexico she had grown up copying the film and TV stars' hairstyles, clothes, and makeup, and she learns a destructive lesson from these shows: "To suffer for love is good. The pain all sweet somehow" ("Hollering," 45).[24] She adopts the language of romance and self-effacement that she learns from the television, displacing any language of agency she may have had. This language becomes the primary structuring device for Cleófilas's reality:

> What Cleófilas has been waiting for, has been whispering
> and sighing and giggling for, has been anticipating since
> she was old enough to lean against the window displays of
> gauze and butterflies and lace, is passion . . . the kind the
> books and songs and *telenovelas* describe when one finds,
> finally, the great love of one's life, and does whatever one
> can, must do, at whatever the cost. ["Hollering," 44]

For Cleófilas, the cost becomes figured in her fascination with the nearby arroyo, La Gritona, or Woman Hollering Creek. The arroyo contains only a trickle of water, and "no one could say whether the woman had hollered from anger or pain" ("Hollering," 46). Cleófilas's puzzlement with the name is met with indifference by her women friends (two of her nearest neighbors are named, incidentally, Dolores and Soledad—pain and loneliness). When she rides in the car with her husband and crosses the bridge, she wonders, "Pain or rage?" and comments to herself that it is "such a funny name for a creek so pretty and full of happily ever after" ("Hollering," 47).

After the first silencing blow from her husband, Cleófilas quickly catapults out of her illusion of happiness: "It left her speechless, motionless, numb. . . . She could think of nothing to say, said nothing. Just stroked the dark curls of the man who wept and would weep like a child, his tears of repentance and shame, this time and each." She endures his drinking parties in the first year of marriage, "sits mute beside their conversation" ("Hollering," 48). In fact, silence becomes a way of life for Cleófilas. Not only is she silenced by her inability to speak English, but her husband's tight control prevents her from phoning or writing her family. Still the language of the *telenovelas* dominates her imagination, and when her husband is away, she sneaks off to Soledad's house, where she watches the shows with her friend.

When he is home, however, Cleófilas also carefully watches her husband, whose fists "at any given moment" would "try to speak" ("Hollering," 48). The language of the fists—"a crack in the face"— adds to silence and shatters Cleófilas's dream of romantic love ("Hollering," 53). Without her own TV set, Cleófilas turns to romance novels to keep the fraying dream alive. When her husband throws one of them at her and it raises a welt on her cheek, it is as if the novel has figuratively turned against her, leaving its mark where her husband's hand usually does. In this incident, Cleófilas begins to realize that her life is, indeed, just like a *telenovela*, as she had wished, "only now the episodes got sadder and sadder. And there were no commercials in between for comic relief. And no happy ending in sight" ("Hollering," 52–53).

Returning from the hospital after giving birth, Cleófilas finds traces of another woman's presence in her home, "a washed cup set back on the shelf wrong-side up. . . . Smudged fingerprint on the door. Crushed cigarette in a glass. Wrinkle in the brain crumpling to a crease" ("Hollering," 50). She doubts herself and tries to believe that her husband's accusations of overexaggeration might be true, but what continues to haunt her are the news reports and her growing fear of him: "This woman found on the side of the interstate. This one pushed from a moving car. This one's cadaver, this one unconscious, this one beaten blue. Her ex-husband, her husband, her lover, her father, her brother, her uncle, her friend, her co-worker. Always" ("Hollering," 52). Like the "slender hair of her doubt," the news corroborates her as-yet unarticulated fear and the very real trajectory of her domestic life.

Threaded through the story like a counterpoint to Cleófilas's silence is the image of the nearly dry Woman Hollering Creek, which fills only when spring comes and it becomes "a good-size alive thing, a thing with a voice all its own, all day and all night calling in its high silver voice." In effect, the creek gives voice when Cleófilas cannot; but its presence is never far from her consciousness, and her musings on it become figures for her own state of mind: "Is it La Llorona, the weeping woman? La Llorona, who drowned her own children. Perhaps La Llorona is the one they named the creek after, she thinks. . . . La Llorona calling to her. She is sure of it. . . . Listens. . . . La Llorona. Wonders if something as quiet as this drives a woman to the darkness under the trees" ("Hollering," 51).[25] Like the articulate and silencing fists of her husband, the creek, figured as a weeping woman, becomes a kind of beckoning language, calling to her, but calling her into a sure madness born of abuse and stultification. As Gloria Anzaldúa argues, La Llorona weeps as an "Indian, Mexican and Chicana's feeble protest when she has no other recourse."[26] Not until she discovers an alternative way of thinking about the creek does Cleófilas turn toward a language of resistance and liberation.

Before that happens, however, Cleófilas becomes pregnant again and tells her husband that she must go to the doctor. Her husband is reluctant but relents when she swears to a code of secrecy, that she would "say she fell down the front steps," assuring him that she would not "make [him] ashamed" ("Hollering," 53). While Cleófilas promises complicity with her husband, her wounds themselves speak when, at the clinic, the nurse reads the language of bruises on her body.[27] Cleófilas's tears clear the space where the old language dies and a new discourse has the possibility of emerging. Unlike the totalizing screams and ultimate silence Scarry describes through torture's unmaking of language, Cleófilas's tears mark the emergence of a new language that washes away silence, secrecy, and collusion. Because of Cleófilas's tears, her body's marks, and her willingness to move out of isolation, the nurse, Graciela, who contacts her friend Felice, takes Cleófilas in hand. Felice, as part of a network of *compañeras* who work with battered women, functions as a reverse *coyote*, one who guides her (quickly, while Cleófilas's husband is at work) across the border back *into* Mexico, and she does so without payment.

Felice startles Cleófilas by meeting her in a pickup truck. ("She herself had chosen it. She herself was paying for it.") But when Felice suddenly hollers "as loud as any mariachi" as they drive across the arroyo, something awakens within Cleófilas. Felice says she does that every time she crosses that bridge. " 'Because of the name, you know. Woman Hollering. *Pues,* I holler. . . . Did you ever notice,' Felice continued, 'how nothing around here is named after a woman? Really. Unless she's the Virgin. I guess you're only famous if you're a virgin. . . . That's why I like the name of that *arroyo.* Makes you want to holler like Tarzan, right?' " ("Hollering," 55). Thus Cleófilas makes an all-important crossing with Felice, who along with Graciela, shatters the *telenovela* images that so define Cleófilas's sense of reality. It is no accident that she turns from Soledad (loneliness) and Dolores (pain) to Graciela (*gracia,* grace) and Felice (*felicidad,* happiness). As a result, Cleófilas hears herself laugh, a kind of laughter not unlike the sound of the full creek in spring, "gurgling out of her own throat, a long ribbon of laughter, like water" ("Hollering," 56), marking a birth out of weeping. She has learned "to decode a feminist message of survival in the haunted voice of the creek that hollers with the rage of a silenced woman."[28] The woman of the creek is not, after all, La Llorona, who drives women to their destruction, but a force—La Gritona—that gives rise to what is almost a war whoop, the emergence of a new and resisting language of liberating joy.

Bebe Moore Campbell creates a densely packed plot and constellation of characters in *Your Blues Ain't Like Mine,* and her themes include the role of poverty and racism in domestic violence. But in this instance the domestic violence occurs within the crucible of a poor white family—the Coxes—that lives just across the garbage-dump border from the community's black sharecroppers and field workers.[29] This proximity, both physical and symbolic, raises the stakes for the Cox family, and brutality becomes not only a way of life but a way of maintaining a phantasmic and radically unstable gender and racial identity. Because the actual power of the Cox men is so tenuous, the exercise of brutality—much as Scarry argues the exercise of torture does for the state—shores up the illusion of power and superiority. Setting this novel in the 1950s through the 1980s, Campbell is clear that race, class, and gender are inextricably linked to the perceived need for power and the battering that exists within Floyd and Lily Cox's home.[30]

After she married Floyd when she was sixteen, Lily quit school, even though she had been a good student ("she was married and she and mama agreed that going back to school didn't make no sense at all" [*Blues*, 15]). The isolation Lily experiences—the loss of friends and the disconnection with everyone but Floyd's family—is not unlike that of Cisneros's Cleófilas. As Lily's life becomes more and more circumscribed, she also resorts to romantic fantasy. Too poor to afford a TV, she watches it on the infrequent visits to a department store where she could "look at *I Love Lucy* and slip into the world of the Ricardos, momentarily forgetting who she was. . . . She wanted to have red, red lips and a bow mouth, to be silly and forever rescued from any predicament" (*Blues*, 124). Lily lives in a world of daydreams and makes do with an occasional tube of lipstick or, in one instance, even a bottle of cologne. But her desire for material things shames Floyd in the face of his poverty. His shame is compounded by the knowledge of his father's and older brother's quiet disapproval of his perceived lack of manliness.

> Floyd remembered the first time Lily saw that bed with the doll on it, the hungry, aching look on her face, as if her cheek would break into tiny shards of glass if he touched it.

> And when she walked into the new bathroom John Earl
> had put in, the naked longing in her eyes felt the same as
> her spitting on him. When they got back to their house, he
> hit her for the first time, smacked her across her porcelain
> cheek with his open palm when she told him that it was
> too cold to walk to the outhouse. "Ain't what I give you
> good enough?" he'd screamed. [*Blues*, 52]

Floyd's violence does its work, and Lily begins silencing herself.
When having sex, she wants to "cry out, to tell him to stop, that
nothing he was doing felt good, but she kept quiet, realizing that her
power [to manipulate him] was gone, that she would have to . . . go
numb" (*Blues*, 11). Although Floyd increasingly asserts himself with
his fists, without him Lily feels "frightened and weak" and as though
she does not exist when he is absent. Lily works hard to keep the
peace with Floyd, hushing the children, making food for him when he
wants it, acquiescing to his sexual demands, and most perniciously,
colluding in the racist lies Floyd tells to protect himself from prosecu-
tion after he commits a murder. In effect, Floyd's language— white
racist and patriarchal discourse—supersedes and silences Lily's own.

The early morning songs and spirituals of the field workers from
the Pinochet plantation haunt and comfort Lily "until her head [is]
full of [them]" and the music applies its soothing balm to her isolation. It is a counterfeit comfort, however. These songs are the cry and
resistance of the field workers and are not hers, something she must
know instinctively, since she feels "lonely and adrift" when the singing stops (*Blues*, 9). Like Precious and Cleófilas, Lily must attempt to
find her own song, her own way of resisting the silencing fist of
domestic violence. But Lily is a spectator borrowing an ephemeral
happiness from others' pain, a pain she reproduces through her collusion in racism. When bored, she longs for exoticism, for a glimpse of
"the Chinaman and his family who ran the town's laundry and
Chinese restaurant. Or maybe the Jew who owned the small department store" (*Blues*, 13). The fetishized Other becomes the magnet for
Lily's fantasies and desire, and the consequences are disastrous when

she wanders into Floyd's pool hall, hears fifteen-year-old Armstrong Todd speaking a few French words, and steps across the line to share a laugh with him. ("The look in her eyes said that she'd done it, had the drink and not gotten caught.") Floyd is embarrassed and outraged when Jake, his employee, later tells him that Armstrong had been "talking [French] to your wife" (*Blues*, 19). His fragile sense of manhood at stake, Floyd is terrified that his father and brother will find out about the incident and, moreover, will discover that he had not sought revenge. At home, terror turns to fury as Floyd beats Lily: "The slap caught her by surprise; it was heavy-handed and so full of meanness and rage she couldn't even cry" (*Blues*, 22).

He cannot stop with simply beating Lily, however. Floyd's shame when his father and brother confront and taunt him leads him to perform a spectacle of white manhood, beating and finally killing Armstrong Todd. Attempting simultaneously to kill the shame he feels and to win acceptance from his father and brother who look on, Floyd screams, "I hate niggers!" when he finally pulls the trigger on Armstrong. Lily depends on popular romantic images (and her necessary sense of herself as a "real" woman—one who has no agency) to justify what Floyd has done: "I got a man who'll kill for me" (*Blues*, 121). In refusing to name Floyd's brutality against her, Lily also becomes complicit in refusing to name the crime Floyd has committed against Armstrong. Instead, she coats it with the lie of male gallantry and dependent womanhood. Lily silences her inquietude about the murder by believing her own lie that Armstrong "assaulted" her womanhood and by telling herself, "Niggers been getting their butts whipped ever since time began; what difference will one more make?"

> Floyd was good to her. Hadn't he bought her the Rio Red lipstick, a scarf, and a bottle of Evening in Paris cologne just to please her. If she didn't have Floyd, what would she do? Her mother and father had passed, her two brothers had moved to Detroit. She hugged herself to keep from shaking, then squeezed his shoulders to reassure herself that he was with her, that he'd always take care of her. . . .

> Well, she knew one thing: There was no telling what that
> [Armstrong] might have done if Floyd hadn't come along
> and saved her. [*Blues*, 47]

The exchange of sexual favors and obedience for a bottle of perfume
and imagined protection is bound to the images of white southern
womanhood that Lily has absorbed and internalized. Lily's perceived
dependence on Floyd is the engine that keeps her lies alive.

But there is a countervailing force, one that causes Lily no small
amount of discomfort. She has, over time, developed a relationship
with an African American woman, Ida Long, who is part of Armstrong Todd's extended family. Lily would occasionally sit in the
"whites only" section of the train station bench, and Ida in the
"colored only" section, and the two would talk, carefully at first,
about their lives. When Ida tells Lily one day that she wants to travel
to Chicago, Lily is astounded, not only by Ida's dream, but that she
actually envied Ida. ("She don't hafta have no husband telling her
what to do.") "The idea, audacious and unspeakable, sparkled before
her as bright as a Christmas ornament. She almost put her hands on
the girl, almost asked her how she got to be like that, to think like
that, but she stopped herself when she realized that she was standing
there envying a colored person" (*Blues*, 32). When Ida tells Lily that
her real father is a white man, Lily in turn tells Ida about her Uncle
Charlie, who "had him a baby by a colored woman." Lily then goes a
step further and tells her that this same uncle also sexually abused
her when she was a little girl and that her mother whipped her for
lying when she reported it to her. As Ida's tears for Lily begin to fall,
Lily takes her in her arms and guiltily tells her about the incident
with Armstrong Todd that had just happened that day, and Ida flees in
a panic. Into that fragile and radical space where the two women
cross racial boundaries, Lily's racism—and indeed the racist system
in which she is complicit—intrudes and ruptures the potential for the
two women to have a healing encounter with each other. While a
flicker of possibility exists in the relationship between Lily and Ida, it

is snuffed out under the system of racial oppression by which both women are constrained, although in quite different ways.

In court for Floyd's trial, Lily finds herself enjoying the attention, and much as Cleófilas had immersed herself in the romance of *telenovelas*, she revels in the sense that she is in a movie, indeed is the *star* of the movie. In court Lily perjures herself ("He—he started saying nasty things to me. Horrible things" [*Blues*, 119]) and conflates what did not happen in Armstrong's presence with the sexual abuse she suffered as a child ("Somewhere in that vision was her uncle Charlie and his probing finger, as murderous as any weapon" [*Blues*, 120]). The entrenched racist system, buttressed by Lily's lies, makes possible the easy acquittal Floyd is given by the all-white jury.

When Lily begins to question her construction of reality, she quickly interdicts herself. "Sometimes she didn't understand men, not even her own husband. She thought about what Floyd had said—that a man had a right to protect his property, his wife, and his kids—and the order of the words struck her. She thought that the way he said it made it seem that she and Floyd junior belonged to him same as if he'd bought and paid for them. *I won't think about that*, she told herself" (*Blues*, 73; emphasis in original). Floyd's abuse of Lily escalates as economic pressures grow (the black community boycotts Floyd's pool hall and effectively closes it down). He beats her regularly, always blaming the beatings somehow on her. When Floyd is sent to Parchman Prison on a later theft charge, this is but the beginning of a string of incarcerations and an ever-progressing alcoholism. Released from prison, he beats and abuses Lily as they move more deeply into desperate poverty. Floyd's beatings silence Lily more and more, and she becomes afraid to ask him for anything. ("He hit her again to make her stop shaking, and again to shut her up" [*Blues*, 140].)

Alone with her two children most of the time, however, and begging for food, Lily finally goes to the welfare department, where her caseworker sodomizes her before issuing a check. Lily's consequent depression and breakdown are not surprising, given her brutalization at the hands of her uncle, her husband, and finally, when she is particularly vulnerable, the welfare caseworker. Silence cracks apart as Lily looks in vain for the bottle of Midnight in Paris, weeps, and then screams with rage, thinking— lucidly—that she "should have started screaming a long time ago" (*Blues*, 235). Somewhat like Tayo's liberating breakdown in *Ceremony*, Lily's scream signals a healing fracture of denial and lies, the beginning of resistance, a road out of her oppression, and she momentarily becomes the unloosed "woman hollering creek" of Cisneros's story. Although hospitalized for a while as she moves from figurative silence to the screaming, Lily finally gives voice, inarticulate as it is, to her pain and rage.

Much as it was with Cleófilas, Lily moves forward only with the help of other women. At first it is Lily's courageous daughter, Doreen, who intervenes when Floyd beats Lily. At one time Doreen pounds on him: "Don't you hit my mother, you jailbird asshole." Lily is speechless. "She had never in her life thought of defending herself against Floyd and watching her teenage daughter fighting for her, she was so overcome that she drifted into a daze and came to life only when Floyd tried to throw Doreen to the ground." When Doreen tells him she will call his parole officer if he ever touches her mother again, "Floyd's face [becomes] pale," and Lily realizes that he is afraid of Doreen, an idea that is "so astounding, so expansive, that Lily's mind couldn't contain it." That night Doreen protectively shares a bed with Lily, "curv[ing] her slim body around the older woman," as Lily thinks again, "He's afraid of her. A girl" (*Blues*, 268), and unlike the counterfeit comfort of the field workers' songs, this very real thought is "as soothing as an old-fashioned swing, rocking her into a sound, peaceful sleep" (*Blues*, 269).

The community of women who help Lily move toward freedom do so indirectly and through Doreen. After Doreen's divorce from her own abusive husband, she and her two daughters convince Lily to leave Floyd and live with them in their trailer. Working at the New Plantation fish plant, Doreen begins organizing with the other women workers, the leader of whom is Lily's onetime almost-friend, Ida. The New Plantation is almost as exploitive as the antebellum southern plantations had been, and as the women workers tell their stories to one another and together analyze their situation (in a model that recalls Paulo Freiere's *conscientização*),[31] they find means to resist the oppressive system. When Lily expresses concern that Doreen is organizing *and* socializing with black women, Doreen exposes the lie of racism and its divisive consequences to poor blacks and whites alike: "I ain't scared of being raped by Willie Horton, Mama. I'm scared of not having medical benefits" (*Blues*, 325). Bringing home to Lily the women's collective wisdom and the fruits of Ida's leadership, Doreen becomes the means for Lily's continued move out of the silence of deception into liberating action. Indeed, when Floyd comes back repeatedly for Lily, she resists, even loading a gun to use on him if necessary, so that she will never be afraid again.

In Sapphire's *Push*, a young woman from Harlem moves out of nearly inchoate trauma into a space of narrative possibility through the process of learning to read and write. Moreover, she does this learning within the liberating context of a community of other young women. In so doing, Precious Jones and her classmates engage in a moral act of listening and telling stories that dismantles the official racist discourse about them, and they create new languages of resistance and health. In storytelling, Arthur Frank notes, "each, teller and listener, enters the space of the story *for* the other. Telling stories in postmodern times, and perhaps in all times, attempts to change one's own life by affecting the lives of others."[32] Before stories can be told and written, language must be found to tell them, however. Both the spoken and the written word will become for Precious the means of powerful resistance as she struggles to find her voice through the community of women who learn to read and write together in an alternative school. In this community, Precious acquires the new, politicized language Ann Russo calls for. With this, she begins to engage her world as a powerful, speaking, writing woman of agency.

But the journey is long and uphill. A neighbor calls 911 after hearing twelve-year-old Precious's screams as she is simultaneously giving birth and being beaten by her mother. After the paramedics arrive, Precious hears the word that will reappear throughout the text like a leitmotif: "Precious, it's almost here. I want you to push. You hear me momi, when that shit hit you again, go with it and push, Preshecita. *Push*" (*Push*, 10).[33] *Push* brings to life the complicated and seemingly intractable issues confronting a survivor of domestic violence and sexual abuse who also struggles against the added systematic assault of racism and poverty.

Predictably, Precious has struggled a great deal in school. In fact, she has completed nine grades of schooling, although she was held back twice—once for the pregnancy and earlier because she could not read ("and I still peed on myself"). In ninth grade she still cannot read, although she desperately wants to. Her desire to learn, however, is eclipsed by the shame of not knowing how to do it (and the consequent show of bravado and disinterest to hide the shame). When a teacher receives no response after asking her to read and repeats the request, Precious responds, "Motherfucker I ain't deaf!" (*Push*, 4). At the same time, however, Precious fantasizes having a "break through" so that she can "learn, catch up, be normal, change my seat to the front of the class." Each day she is forced, however, to admit, "it has not been that day" (*Push*, 5). Precious, like Zora Neale Hurston's famous character Janey Crawford, has an inside and an outside and "knows not to mix them."[34] Precious's schooling reaches a crisis when she is finally thrown out for being pregnant with her second child ("You can't suspend me for being pregnant, I got rights!" [*Push*, 8]).

It is no surprise that Precious has been unable to learn. Life at home is a nightmare, and the school system is ill prepared to work with such a child. Her mother weighs more than 300 pounds and has not left the house in five years; she depends on Precious for physical survival and even sexual gratification. When her mother's rage becomes uncontrollable, she batters Precious. In addition, her father, Carl, began raping her when she was in diapers and continued throughout her childhood. ("I see me, first grade, pink dress dirty sperm stuffs on it. No one comb my hair. Second grade, third grade, fourth grade seem like one dark night. Carl is the night and I disappear in it.") Sapphire clearly links Precious's difficulties in school to the abuse. Indeed, after she has been beaten or raped, "Don't make sense talking, bouncing balls, filling in between dotted lines. Shape? Color? Who care whether purple shit a square or a circle, whether it purple or blue?" (*Push*, 18). Tests ("tesses") come back telling Precious she has "no brain." "The tesses paint a picture of me an' my muver—my whole family, we more than dumb, we invisible" (*Push*, 30).

Not unlike Pecola Breedlove, Precious experiences what Beth E. Richie calls "gender entrapment," a phenomenon in which black women's "problems are blamed on individual character flaws: women are considered masochistic, with self-defeating personality disorders, confused in their decision-making, unable to solve serious problems."[35] Perhaps one of Precious's most important utterances at the beginning of the novel is the line, "There is something wrong with the tesses." In it exist the seeds of her resistance that will lead her to a new sense of agency as she learns new narratives, new ways of speaking and writing about her reality. But until she does, Precious's narrative is one of invisibility and rage.

> I big, I talk, I eats, I cooks, I laugh, watch TV, do what my muver say. But I can see when the picture come back I don't exist. Don't nobody want me. Don't nobody need me. I know who I am. I know who they say I am—vampire sucking the system's blood. Ugly black grease to be wipe away, punish, kilt, changed, finded a job for. . . . I wanna say I am somebody. I wanna say it on subway, TV, movie, LOUD. I see the pink faces in suits look over top of my head. I watch myself disappear in their eyes, their tesses. I talk loud but still I don't exist. [*Push*, 31]

Sapphire links Precious's sense of invisibility and dissociation both to the abuse she endures at the hands of her father and mother and to the social context of poverty and racism in which the whole family is caught. The suffering Precious endures is intense. After being raped, she would often cut herself with a razor and rub feces on her face, performing and mirroring the pain and humiliation of the rape: "I am a TV set wif no picture. I am broke wif no mind. No past or present time. Only the movies of being someone else . . . a pink virgin girl" (*Push*, 112).

After a social worker's visit, Precious reluctantly looks into the alternative school the social worker recommended. Knowing that the social worker has a "file" on her infuriates Precious, and when she finds out that it has been sent to the school, her fury is doubled. The file becomes a figure for Precious's disempowerment by the systems and institutions within which she struggles simply to survive (school, welfare, hospital/medical). Despite her anger, her desire to learn triumphs, and Precious decides to try the school. When she enters the room, she sees a half-dozen other young women and a teacher with "long dreadlocky hair" and becomes terrified that she will wet herself as she did in the second grade. Her instinct for survival pushes Precious to stay in the room, however, and for the first time in her life, she chooses to resist the educational script of failure that has been written for her (and thousands like her) throughout the ages: "The whole class quiet. Everybody staring at me. God don't let me cry. I takes air in through my nose, a big big breath, then I start to walk slow to the back. But something like birds or light fly through my heart. An' my feet stop. At the first row. An' for the first time in my life I sits down in the front row (which is good 'cause I never could see the board from the back)" (*Push*, 40). In this moment, Precious senses that she will "kill [herself] first" before she will ever sit in the back again.

Precious's teacher, Blue Rain, is, as Cheryl Clarke describes, "the Shug Avery of adult basic education" and, much like Alice Walker's character in *The Color Purple*, is both healer and inspiriting presence. When Blue Rain asks her if she feels she is in the right place,

> I want to tell her what I always wanted to tell someone, that the pages, 'cept for the ones with pictures, look all the same to me; the back row I'm not in today; how I sit in a chair seven years old all day wifout moving. But I'm not

seven years old. But I am crying. I look Miz Rain in the
face, tears is coming down my eyes, but I'm not sad or em-
barrass. [*Push*, 48]

Precious's teacher works with the students to create a learning community through daily reading, writing, and storytelling. They begin
by writing sounds and copying the alphabet in their notebooks. Blue
Rain asks the women to write what is on their minds, even though
they might not know how to spell it. For Precious, this experience is
"music in [her] head." Precious begins by writing in her journal, "li
Mg o mi m" (little Mongo [her first child, who has Down's syndrome]
on my mind). Rain's response below Precious's line, "Who is Little
Mongo?" thus begins a written dialogue that will continue until it
blossoms into Precious's own poetry and prose. One's own work is
never created in isolation. It is the context of Precious's learning that
is so important. Blue Rain and the students create a classroom of
collaboration and community. They learn to read and write with the
raw and painful materials of their lives. As they share more and more
details of their stories with one another, they become bearers both of
testimony and of witness, sharing in the difficult business of uncover-
ing truth and the language to tell it.

The sense of joy Precious feels when she reads an entire line ("I
want to cry. I want to laugh. I want to hug and kiss Miz Rain. She
make me feel good. I never reading nuffin' before" [*Push*, 54–55])
leads to other profound changes in her behavior and thinking. Like
Celie, also in *The Color Purple*, Precious makes a shift away from a
paralyzing, other-directed rage to an inner-directed love.[36] For example, when she has disturbing nightmares about being abused by her
mother and father and feels like killing them, she shifts the focus to
herself. "I call little Precious and say, Come to Mama but I means me.
Come to *me* little Precious. Little Precious look at me, smile, and start
to sing: ABCDEFG" (*Push*, 59). On her birthday Precious lights a
candle for herself: "I glad Precious Jones was born. I like baby I
born. It gets to suckes from my bress" (*Push*, 68). Adding the poster
of Harriet Tubman given to her by Ms. Rain to the one she already

has of Louis Farrakhan, Precious tells her baby, Abdul Jamal Louis Jones, "Listen, baby, Muver love you. Muver not dumb. Listen baby: ABCDEFGHIJKLMNOPQRSTUVWXYZ" (*Push*, 66).

With self-love and self-respect comes the power to resist the destructive rage that has prevented her from learning. In addition, however, Precious learns to resist even those who love her. When Blue Rain suggests that Precious give Abdul up for adoption, she adamantly refuses, struggling to stay in school even when her mother, in a jealous rage, tries to kill her and throws her out of the house after she returns from the hospital. After experiencing a night of chaos in a shelter, she goes straight to Ms. Rain, who is outraged at what has happened ("she mumbling and cursing about *what* damn safety net, most basic needs, a newborn child, A NEWBORN CHILD! She going OFF now" [*Push*, 78]).

Finding a place in a halfway house, Precious continues her schooling and works with new students as they join the class ("You know how you write to teacher 'n she write back to you in the same journal book like you talkin' on paper and you could SEE your talk coming back to you when the teacher answer you back" [*Push*, 94]). As Gayle Pemberton points out, "For Precious . . . fiction and poetry are the means toward finding a tenable vision of [herself]."[37] By now Precious owns eight books, including Ann Petry's work about Harriet Tubman, Arnold Adoff's *Malcolm X*, Walker's *The Color Purple*, and Langston Hughes's ("the dream keeper!") selected poems. Abdul also has his own books, two by Lucille Clifton and others by Ezra Jack Keats, Monique Felix, and Crokett Johnson. Precious memorizes and recites for the class Langston Hughes's poem "Mother to Son," affirming to herself that "life for me ain't been no crystal stair" (*Push*, 112–13). As Precious grows intellectually and as a mother, she revises the myth of the welfare queen most of white society believes with stunning persistence, "the lazy mother on public assistance who deliberately breeds children at the expense of taxpayers to fatten her monthly check."[38]

Precious falls in love with *The Color Purple*, identifying with Celie's suffering and emergence, and adds Walker's poster to Tubman's and Farrakhan's. Farrakhan's insistence on black pride, Tubman's efforts to free slaves, and Walker's affirmation of personal change and growth all stand in mimetic relation to Precious's own processes of empowerment and liberation. Precious insists to the class that she loves Celie, "except I ain' no butch," since her other hero, Farrakhan, has denounced homosexuality.[39] Shocked by Blue's disclosure that she is a lesbian, within seconds Precious shifts allegiances and declares, "Too bad about Farrakhan." Precious comes to understand that "homos not who rape me, not homos who let me sit up not learn for sixteen years, not homos who sell crack fuck Harlem. . . . Ms Rain the one who put the chalk in my hand, make me queen of the ABCs" (*Push*, 81). Precious's poetry soon begins to express love for her lesbian teacher:

> Blu Ran
> Blue RAIN
> Rain
> Is gr——
> (gray)
> but saty
> (stay)
> my rain. [*Push*, 90]

Despite her adoration of Ms. Rain, Precious learns to disagree with her, thus clearing space for her own articulated critique. For example, when Rain brings up the "problem" of *The Color Purple*'s fairy-tale ending, Precious thinks, "Sometimes I wanna tell Ms Rain shut up with all the IZM stuff. But she my teacher so I don't tell her shut up. I don't know what 'realism' mean but I do know what REALITY is and it's a mutherfucker, lemme tell you" (*Push*, 83). She also learns that such reality is not limited to poor African American women, as she reads about a white woman whose husband beats her and about the many women who exist in living hells across class and racial lines. She adds another important word to her vocabulary: "battery."

After discovering that her father has transmitted HIV to her (but not, thankfully, to Abdul), Precious is devastated and believes she will never write again:

> Hammer in my heart now, beating me, I feel like my blood
> a giant river swell up inside me and I'm drowning. My
> head all dark inside. Feel like giant river I never cross in
> front of me now. Ms Rain say, You not writing Precious. I
> say I drownin' in river. She don't look me like I'm crazy
> but say, If you just sit there the river gonna rise up drown
> you! Writing could be the boat carry you to the other side.
> One time in your journal you told me you had never really
> told your story. I think telling your story git you over that
> river Precious. . . . "I'm tired," I says. She says, "I know
> you are but you can't stop now Precious, you gotta push."
> And I do. [*Push*, 96– 97]

As Precious pushes herself to write, she encounters another layer of rage within herself ("I think I AM / MAD / ANGERREEY angerry / very / mi life / not good" [*Push*, 100]). Learning more about what has happened to her, she adds another word to her political vocabulary: "incest." She writes prolifically, working out her anger and fear on paper.

At the urging of one of her classmates, she eventually attends a support group for incest survivors and is amazed that what she has read in books only scratches the surface of what many women have suffered. "It's all kinda girls here! They sitting in circle faces like clocks, no bombs. Bombs with hair and titties and dresses. After I sit here five minutes I know I am a bomb too. Only sitting here doing whatever they gonna do will keep me from blowing up. Thank you Rita for git me here on time" (*Push*, 129). When she speaks for the first time, she raises her hand and, in that gesture, actively reverses the experience of torture, taking the inchoate silence of her victimization and giving it words of resistance: "My hand is going up through the smell of Mama, my hand is pushing Daddy's dick out my face." She begins to wonder beyond her own experience as she hears what others have endured: "What kinda world this babies raped. A father break a girl's arm. . . . All kinda women here. Princess girls, some fat girls, old women, young women. One thing we got in common, no *the* thing, is we was rape" (*Push*, 130).

Precious's expanding worldview is evident in her writing as she takes as her themes the streets of Harlem and life outside herself, becoming both critical and appreciative of what she sees. Although Precious's reading scores are too low to pass the General Educational Development (GED) test, she knows and is further affirmed by Ms. Rain that she is "passionate." Precious also believes that "can't no numbers measure how far I done come in jus' two years" (*Push*, 108). Her reading scores being what they are, however, Precious becomes suspicious of the social worker's questions and one day steals her file from the office. With the help of one of her classmates, Precious reads the entire file. She becomes outraged when she sees that the social worker notes that her scores are "disappointingly low" ("Not to Ms Rain! Not to Ms Rain!" [*Push*, 118]) and that "in keeping with the new initiative on welfare reform," she should enter a work-fare program. "Despite her obvious intellectual limitations she is quite capable of working as a home attendant" (*Push*, 119). Intervening in her own officially charted story, Precious resists the racist discourse ("all she see for me is wiping ol white people's ass" [*Push*, 121]) that structures and underlies welfare reform. She insists on getting her GED, along with a job "and a place for [herself] and Abdul, then . . . college" (*Push*, 120). Precious understands that living in a white person's house as an "attendant" means getting paid for eight hours a day and that the other sixteen would be akin to slavery. She names it and writes it: "slavery." She knows that she would see Abdul only on Sundays and, doing the math, figures that with pay of $3.35 an hour she would actually earn $1.12 an hour with that kind of setup. Precious resists by reading the chart and—at no small risk to herself— heroically constructs a narrative of resistance.

She continues to revise the narrative as she confronts her mother, who tries to blame Precious for the abuse she suffered and survived at home ("I think she some kind of freak baby" [*Push*, 136]). After the session, Precious is sad, but so full of herself: "I think how *alive* I am, every part of me that is cells, proteens, nutrons, hairs, pussy, eyeballs, nervus sistem, brain. I got poems, a son, friends. I want to live so bad" (*Push*, 137). For her, resistance and the emergence of a politicized language lead to a capacious and loving worldview, a spiritual awakening: "I see those men in vacant lot share one hot dog and they homeless, that's good as Jesus with his fish. I remember when I had my daughter [Little Mongo], nurse nice to me—all that is god. Shug in *Color Purple* say it's the 'wonder' of purple flowers. I feel that, even though I never seen or had no flowers like what she talk about" (*Push*, 139). Reading and writing give Precious back her life as she has struggled to regain it within community(s) of women who search for the same. She is still infected with HIV and is still coping with poverty and the appalling lack of resources for single mothers. The novel ends with the presentation of a "Class Book," which contains the equally horrific and triumphant stories of Precious's classmates. As Cheryl Clarke says, "Telling the stories is never enough," and "we learn . . . that the atrocities are as infinite as the stories that recount them."[40]

Just as Precious rises out of the ashes of abuse and illiteracy to name the horrors that she has experienced and to transform her life, Cleófilas learns to turn weeping into laughter, moving from the isolation of her trauma into articulating it with her body's bruises to the health care worker (who is well-enough connected in the community to find someone to take Cleófilas away from her situation). As Cleófilas finds language to name the creek, she also finds within herself the power to begin resisting. Lily finally learns to say no, loading a gun and refusing to be afraid of her husband again. This move is made through the stuttered rising of truth within her but, moreover, through the solidarity she finds with her daughter and the knowledge her daughter brings to her from organizing with other women to fight injustice. Marked first by screams of rage, Lily's growing power to resist evolves as she listens to the truth that is within her, as she displaces silence and lies with the language of truth. All three characters emerge from a nearly wordless experience of violence into a liberated—and healing—space by way of language, naming, and loving community. These are ragged spaces, however; as work that looks at recovery from sexual trauma suggests, healing is not a simple trajectory, nor is it ever completed.

All three of the texts discussed in this chapter suggest that since voice is such an important aspect of healing, making the space for the emergence of that voice is an important role medicine can play beyond the bandaging of wounds. Paying attention, learning to identify the symptoms and signs of battering and sexual abuse is a start. For example, after training and protocols on domestic violence were introduced at the Medical College of Pennsylvania, the proportion of female trauma patients identified by clinicians as battered increased dramatically from 5.6 to 30 percent.[41] Marilynne Bell and Janet Mosher argue that clinicians need to pay attention to "the realities of women's lives."[42] They call for physicians to resist stereotypes and deal with their own assumptions about why women are abused. This might include, for example, being able to challenge a woman who insists that she is powerless to change her situation. They also insist on the importance of leaving behind the security of the biomedical model and accumulating the perspectives and wisdom of those outside, including the woman herself.

When a physician does understand and gives domestic violence a name, however, what resources are available to her or him? As Warshaw says, "What is potentially lethal for any battered woman is not necessarily her current injuries or symptoms but her return home to a situation of escalating violence."[43] In Chicago alone, with 55,000 domestic violence cases in the courts and 8,100 calls on the domestic violence helpline, there were 211 shelter beds available for battered women in 1999. Going beyond treating symptoms is complex—nearly impossible—given the paucity of resources. Without enlightened laws and policies, responsive and capacious institutions, and community support for battered women, the work physicians can do is limited. This does not mean that health care practitioners should continue to treat domestic and sexual violence only symptomatically, but that the community must also bear its share of responsibility in enacting positive social change and supporting just and responsive social structures. Physicians and other health care workers cannot single-handedly effect urgently needed structural and social reforms, but they can and should add their voices to the struggle, becoming well-informed advocates (and adding the good lists of community resources that do exist to their arsenals of technologies and medications). Cisneros, Campbell, and Sapphire insist that health care practitioners consider the multiple social, political, and personal strands that form the pattern of domestic and sexual violence so that they will be partners in helping their patients find, as Lucille Clifton writes, "safe houses, / hands [they] can trust."

There Was Much Left Unexplained

Narrative Complications and Technological Limitations in
Gloria Naylor's *Mama Day* and Ana Castillo's *So Far from God*

6

> Por allá vienen las viudas
> Las madres y las hermanas
>
> There come the widows
> The mothers and the sisters
> —Julia de Burgos, "Ochenta Mil"

> People just don't know the power that black magic have, or root have because
> of the fact it just unbelievable. You have to see it to believe it.
> —Jacie Burns, in *Walkin' over Medicine*

> Doña Julia had embroidered the story like a pattern of vines on a pillowcase;
> the threads were tangled underneath, but on the surface a complex design was
> becoming clear and evident to Doña Tina.
> —Judith Ortiz Cofer, *The Line of the Sun*

Much as the women telling stories in Judith Ortiz Cofer's novel do, Gloria Naylor's and Ana Castillo's characters embroider stories that also have their tangled threads underneath; they are stories that claim truths while they complicate them. Illustrating a shift of focus from that of the authors discussed in the preceding chapters, Naylor and Castillo raise questions of interpretative strategies, peering underneath the realm of the empirical and verifiable, pushing readers to consider the many challenges that representations of illness and healing demand. *Mama Day* and *So Far from God* do not simply ask readers to consider interpretative difficulties, however. As do all of the novels considered in this study, they write themselves against the grain of dominant notions of how the world works, foregrounding aspects of culture that have been erased or denigrated, in this instance and among other things, rootwork and *curandismo*. In addition, both novels employ a mix of humor and magical realism to level

137

a critique at rational, technological, contemporary biomedicine di-vorced from social context and justice. Much as the other novels considered in this book, both *Mama Day* and *So Far from God* embed illness and healing in a social and political context, thus contesting individualistic interpretations of illness that would seek causes and explanatory models primarily within the body (and sometimes the mind) of the patient.[1] Instead, these novels link those illnesses (and injuries) with the social body—the contexts and the communities—from which they emerge.

Mama Day and *So Far from God*, then, seek to reconstruct what has been lost to dominant paradigms about illness, the body, and healing. In so doing, they challenge the hegemony of empiricism as well as seek to dismantle absolute trust in technology. In addition, they map human illness and suffering to their political and social roots. Frantz Fanon's analysis of colonialism illustrates, in part, the reverse mecha-nisms of these novels. "Colonialism is not satisfied merely with hold-ing a people in its grip and emptying the native's brain of all form and content. By a kind of perverted logic, it turns to the past of the oppressed people, and distorts, disfigures, and destroys it."[2] In re-claiming what has been distorted, disfigured, and destroyed, Naylor and Castillo recast such healing practices as rootwork and *curandismo* into powerful and significant forces in the healing (and making ill) of human beings, and in so doing, they contest strictly biomedical expla-nations of health and illness. The novels are thus oppositional; that is, they oppose, challenge, subvert, and revise dominant forms of knowl-edge. The eroding of dominant narratives that occurs in these novels permits a kaleidoscope of truths to emerge, and perhaps less-accepted but more diverse possibilities also emerge. By looking at illness and healing specifically, both novels complicate a historically dominant interpretative enterprise by calling on marginalized, mostly nonveri-fiable, and sometimes just simply mysterious traditions.

It is, of course, something of the human condition and certainly a condition of the practice of medicine to live with uncertainty, mys-tery, and an ultimate sense of unknowability. But the knowledge of uncertainty is frequently lost (or submerged) in the scramble for better technologies and ever more precise measures.[3] Naylor and Castillo resist and complicate what Arthur Frank calls "medical colonization."[4] Frank argues that storytelling among the community of the ill is the primary way of resisting such colonization. But Naylor and Castillo turn medical colonization on its head, invoking what M. M. Bakhtin calls the carnivalesque, a method used not only to laugh at dominant forces within a society but to analyze them: "Laughter has the remarkable power of making an object come up close, of drawing it into a zone of crude contact where one can finger it familiarly on all sides, turn it upside down, inside out, peer at it from above and below, break open its external shell, look into its center, doubt it, take it apart, dismember it, lay it bare and expose it."[5] By employing the carnivalesque, these novels resist the tendency of medicine to colonize illness, and instead they hold medicine at bay, confound its categories, and celebrate the manifold mysteries of healing.[6]

How does institutional medicine deal with mystery? On one hand, a good practitioner will readily admit that healing is frequently beyond the understanding of rational medicine. On the other, practitioners are often reluctant to engage patients in a discussion of their own interpretative frameworks—and for good reason. As these novels demonstrate, the interpretations that some patients may bring to their ailments are nearly indecipherable to modern medicine. In addition, they call on the hearers (those who function, frequently, as witnesses to difficult realities undergirding the narratives of explanation given by their patients) to suspend judgment for a time, much as a fictional narrative might (think of Samuel Taylor Coleridge's claim that a good reader needs a momentary and willing suspension of disbelief). While institutionalized medicine becomes more and more mired in the politics of managed care, many ethicists have begun to call for an approach that turns to narrative—messy and difficult though it may be—as a primary epistemological means in the diagnosis, care, and treatment of patients.

Undermining the primacy of a solely empirical medical epistemology, these stories in their interpretative difficulty suggest that real patients' individual illnesses and traumas are even more complex.

Interpretative frameworks, these novels warn us, are not simple matters. In the last several years, much has been written about an emerging category of biomedical ethics often called narrative ethics or narrative bioethics.[7] The jury is still out as to all that narrative ethics is, but simply put, it can be seen as a means of approaching ethical decision making that relies for its epistemology not on classical abstract categories (beneficence, autonomy, justice, and so forth) but on the narrative context and stories of patient, caregiver, and family/friends.[8] Scholars writing about narrative ethics point out that this less wieldy, inductive method allows for the *possibility* of a more patient-centered approach that is less hierarchical and more interested in getting to the truth (or more accurately, a set of truths) by means of the contexts and "stories" of those involved in the case.[9] Because medical knowledge is uncertain, the practice of narrative ethics, says Kathryn Montgomery Hunter, attempts "to set out accounts of events in order to explore imaginatively their meaning for the people they affect and to determine what action should be taken."[10] In her introduction to an essay of "five stories," Rita Charon states that "the narratives of medicine—from the illness itself, to patients' verbal utterances in medical interviews, to hospital chart entries—must be recognized . . . by listening to them, reading them, or writing them down." Doctors and patients alike must "achieve contextual understandings of singular human experiences, supporting the recognition of multiple contradictory meanings of complex events."[11] Anne Hudson Jones looks at the possibility of a shift in the power balance with the use of narrative: "Nonhierarchical and dialogic in nature, a narrative approach seeks to encourage all those involved in a particular ethical dilemma to become engaged in its resolution. Because ethical decisions must be enacted by persons who are powerfully emotional beings, abstract logic may not be sufficient to achieve the best resolution."[12]

While decision making may not always involve life or death issues, power resides in every decision made regarding one's health care or the understanding of one's illness and healing. Narrative, as a primary epistemological means in medicine, then, extends to actual care of the patient as well as the process of making ethical decisions. In this way, how one gets to the particular decision becomes as important as (and perhaps even more important than) the decision itself. A narrative approach to ethics—at its best—seeks to create space for the silenced (or, as we have seen in Tayo's case, strategically silent). Such an approach helps shift the balance of power from clinicians and hospital officials to patient and family. Moreover, it looks to provide a context where the deeply personal of all those involved is honored. It is a method that has the potential—and I use the word "potential" with care—of placing patients and families in a broader and, perhaps, a more politicized context. As Kathryn Hunter emphasizes, narrative bioethics makes sure questions will be asked and attempts to make room for the understanding that "moral knowledge is inevitably subjective, always open to question, discussion, elaboration, retelling, and reinterpretation."[13] Narrative ethics recognizes the multiple lenses and facets of the interpretative gesture that complicates knowing deliberately by including those multiplicities but, in so doing, acknowledges the profound complexity of human experience.

In many ways, *Mama Day* and *So Far from God* exemplify the thorniness of the interpretative pathways of narrative ethics. Both novels provide readers with unknowable phenomena and often construct multiple stories around those phenomena. The writers make sure that readers eager for the facts will *never* apprehend the whole story. Instead, Naylor and Castillo use uncertainty to critique a kind of textual imperialism that would lead readers to think they know (or could know, if they just worked hard enough) the whole story, one we might believe is ours by rights. This critique of textual imperialism extends, by virtue of the content of the stories, to a medical colonization that would seek to contain and explain all through a narrow, biomedical lens only. In *Mama Day*, Cocoa's husband struggles with his need to reject what he perceives to be backwoods superstition. He wants to seek "expert" medical help rather than listen to Mama Day's and the community's interpretation of what has happened to Cocoa, and it costs him his life. In *So Far from God*, various members of the community of Tome, New Mexico—especially Sofi's realistic (and desperately middle-class) daughter, Fe—fight what they see as ignorant and superstitious beliefs that are grounded in an overzealous religious faith. In addition, the content of both novels consistently raises the question, What is going on? It is a question to which narrative ethics (at its best) applies itself readily through the stories and interpretations of everyone involved.

In addition to confounding neat interpretative strategies, Naylor and Castillo level a critique at an unexamined belief in technology that would seek to find answers and solutions primarily in and through the use of technology. Castillo, in writing about *curandismo*, for example, argues that the basis of modern medicine and medical technology lies in "very ancient practices" that have been lost.[14] These are not Luddite texts, but they do warn readers that, along with the complexities of narrative truths, dependence on and misuse of technology extract a high price—in some cases, the price of a life. For example, corporate and government misuse of technologies created for the military industry, itself a killing machine, causes the death of one of the characters in *So Far from God*. Similarly, George, in *Mama Day*, dies largely as a result of his failure to let go of his faith in technology (and, not coincidentally, himself as a rational, independent male) and to embrace (literally, to take hands with) the values and ways of seeing represented by Mama Day and the Willow Springs community in order to heal Cocoa. The novels call readers to look at truth from a variety of perspectives, truths that elude the biomedical gaze. Additionally, while the novels challenge an absolute faith in contemporary biomedicine, they create models of collaboration, connection, and community accountability from which medicine might profitably learn.

The irrationally jealous Ruby poisons Cocoa in *Mama Day*, but Ruby augments that poison with something (and we never know quite what) that causes maggotlike worms to devour Cocoa from within her body (much as overweening jealousy devours Ruby from within herself). The means to Cocoa's actual healing also remain puzzling when extracted from the realm of allegory (love, self-sacrifice, prayer—but *how* Cocoa actually becomes well is a mystery). Naylor joins Cocoa's story with that of Bernice, who becomes pregnant by a combination of Mama Day's commonsense natural remedies and her use of the suggestion of supernatural power at the "other place," confounding readers' expectations that the form be either allegory (a tidy way to explain the magic or supernatural phenomena) or realistic representation (what is the exact disease? the exact cure? what is going on here?).

Castillo's *So Far from God* similarly defeats such expectations, but it does so even more blatantly (and hilariously). The seriocomic novel presents the tales of a mother, her errant husband, and her four exceptional daughters, beginning with the youngest, who "dies" at age three and is resurrected at her funeral. She flies to the church roof and spends the rest of her life avoiding most human contact (and is also somewhat prescient, foretelling many events). All of the daughters die before the end of the novel, and most of the deaths are related in some way to social and political evils in their worlds. Many of their injuries and/or illnesses are as mysterious as their recoveries and, later, deaths, however.

Both novels thematically raise questions of interpretative strategies and conflict around those interpretations. In *Mama Day*, Cocoa's urbane (and highly rational) husband, George, simply cannot accept the idea that Cocoa's illness and recovery depend on something beyond technological biomedical resources (that are, as a hurricane would have it, not available to Cocoa anyway). Mama Day's and the community's interpretations of what has happened to Cocoa are outrageous to him, and he rejects them out of hand until, driven by desperation, he allows Mama Day to instruct him in what appears to him to be an outlandish activity that he believes bears no relation to his wife dying in her grandmother's house. Similar, although less foregrounded, are various characters' interpretations of events in *So Far from God*. Sofi's conservative daughter, Fe, rationally explains that her sister's flight to the church roof was an illusion borne of the stress of seeing her "come back to life" after what was clearly a serious epileptic seizure. Later in the novel, however, other more or less reliable characters verify the flight story. In more than one instance, a character will voice to her- or himself some private reservation about what appear to be other outlandish stories. In this way, both novels insist that readers think about the act of interpretation itself, showing it as a multifaceted activity that, to be done best, employs a number of vantage points. It is as though both novels rely on Emily Dickinson's advice to "tell the truth but tell it slant," understanding that epistemological success "in circuit lies."[15] Both novels circle truth in ways that disallow neat verification.

Critics have pointed out that Naylor's novel functions both as Christian allegory and as a remake of Shakespeare's *The Tempest.*[16] *Mama Day* takes place in New York City and Willow Springs, a small island off the coast of South Carolina, neither a foreign country nor a territory of the United States. Naylor's novel focuses less on the social conditions that give rise to illness than on what I would call an etiology of hate in the construction of the illness of her main character, Cocoa. *Mama Day*, in creating "a world outside white parameters" and in critiquing George's reliance on white constructs and ways of being, reminds readers that racism, both internal and external, is as deadly as any spell or rootwork done for spite.[17] Castillo's *So Far from God*, however, deliberately situates every ailment (and there are many) in social and political contexts, much as do the other novels in this study. Like *Mama Day*, *So Far from God* critiques white/Anglo constructs and epistemologies (while laughing at them). Both *Mama Day* and *So Far from God* leave ambiguous the causes (and types) of their character's illnesses or wounds and leave equally mysterious the means of their healing.[18]

Both novels bear striking similarities to each other. Each has a central female healer—Mama Day and Doña Felicia (*So Far from God*)—and both novels focus primarily on female communities. Both healers rely on natural herbal remedies, although Doña Felicia is much more overtly grounded than Mama Day in a somewhat unusual Catholic/Christian faith, relying heavily on prayer and the intervention of the saints.[19] While *Mama Day*'s main character, Cocoa, is the novel's primary focus, and it is her serious illness that occupies most of the story, Bernice's conception and delivery of her child also involves intervention by Mama Day and has its own interpretative difficulties. In *So Far from God*, three of Sofi's daughters (Caridad, Fe, and La Loca) are stricken with illness, and Caridad is mysteriously cured. The fourth daughter is murdered as a political prisoner in the Middle East but later returns as a spirit. Each novel has a male "healer" or mystic, and both are slightly off center. Dr. Buzzard, in Naylor's novel, is seen by Mama Day as a pure charlatan who practices a bogus HooDoo to instill fear in the community. In *So Far from God*, Francisco, an ascetic carver of wooden santos, falls in love with Caridad (who herself becomes a healer) and becomes increasingly unhinged until he finally hangs himself. Sofi, the mother, also has her counterpart in *Mama Day*, Cocoa's grandmother who raised her, Abigail Day. There are also physicians in both novels. Dr. Smithfield is from across the bridge and holds Mama Day's powers in high regard. Dr. Tolentino is a family practice doctor who delivers all of Sofi's girls and also has a talent for psychic surgery learned in his homeland, the Philippines. While *Mama Day* has been described as "a virtual encyclopedia of African American expressive culture,"[20] the same could be said for *So Far from God* and southwestern Chicano culture.[21]

Mama Day opens with the figure of an anthropologist ("Reema's boy") returned from the university to study the community and its interpretation of a long-used (and for him and other academics, long-misunderstood) term, "18 & 23," the date Sapphira Wade received her freedom from slavery.[22] In his zeal to see the truth, he misses it completely, writing a book that makes academic sense but is absolute nonsense to the people living in Willow Springs:

> He had come to the conclusion after "extensive field work" (ain't never picked a boll of cotton or head of lettuce in his life—Reema spoiled him silly), but he done still made it to the conclusion that 18 & 23 wasn't 18 and 23 at all—was

> really 81 & 32, which just so happened to be the lines of
> longitude and latitude marking off where Willow Springs
> sits on the map. And we were just so damned dumb that
> we turned the whole thing around. . . . Not that he called it
> being dumb, mind you, called it "asserting our cultural
> identity," "inverting hostile social and political parame-
> ters." [*Mama Day*, 7–8]

In a sense, the scholarly anthropologist functions as a figure for the
diagnostician—one who wants to discover the truth about unknown
phenomena. It is not that the anthropologist is necessarily wrong to
want to know, but that he simply did not talk with the people or,
more important, listen carefully, and that he relied on, or was too
heavily inside of, logical-rational constructs (such as maps). As the
narrator says, "Someone who didn't know how to ask wouldn't know
how to listen" either (*Mama Day*, 10). Similarly the men who want to
develop the island into a "vacation paradise" simply cannot see the
vast spiritual resources of Willow Springs. The novel thus warns
readers early in its pages that an imperialistic approach to its stories
will be doomed to misreading and probable misunderstanding. Stories about Sapphira Wade, for example, the matriarch of the Day
family, resist unitary interpretation. Sapphira Wade is not only a
healer, but she is one who threw the notion of interpretation into
question. "She turned the moon into salve, the stars into a swaddling
cloth, and healed the wounds of every creature walking up on two or
down on four. It ain't about right or wrong, truth or lies; it's about
a slave woman who brought a whole new meaning to both them
words" (*Mama Day*, 3).

From this beginning, readers are invited to share in the construction of knowledge that comes by way of an omniscient narrator and
the conversations between Cocoa and her dead husband, George.
Readers are given a comprehensive history of Mama Day's family
and the events that shaped the lives of each character. This occurs by
way of nonlinear plotting through recall, flashback, and conversation
and becomes a pieced quilt of narrative insight.[23] Much like life

stories, including those told within a medical setting, these are stories that wend their ways, sometimes in a circle, toward understanding the changes within the body due to illness or injury, and the truths of those changes. What readers learn about the stories of each character will help them understand and construct their own interpretative frameworks; but events happen in the novel that simply do not fit rational constructs, and these things have to do with illness, healing, and the body's own knowledge.

Miranda, also known as "Mama Day," has a connection with nature that allows her to read a droplet of water and gain the foreknowledge of her granddaughter's visit. She and her sister, Abigail (Cocoa's grandmother), both understand the ways of natural medicine, but Mama Day ("MD") is the acclaimed healer of the village, having brought many babies into the world and having healed many people of their maladies. She is described as having second sight and "gifted hands." As Lindsay Tucker argues, Mama Day's curative powers stem in particular from her knowledge of conjure, not Santeria, Obeah, or Voodoo (which are all linked to their particular locales). Tucker explains that conjure treats three types of illnesses: "(1) natural illnesses for which a knowledge of roots, herbs, barks, and teas is applied; (2) so-called occult, or spiritually connected, illnesses which require spell casting and charms; and (3) illnesses which include both personal and collective calamities that are not the result of malevolent practices."[24] Mama Day, however, goes far beyond Tucker's categories for conjure, since she clearly deals with an illness that is the result of malevolent practice, Ruby's spell on Cocoa. She is a conjure woman, but she is more.

Another character, Dr. Buzzard, fits more easily into the "world of occult medicine and is clearly the hoodoo doctor described in so many studies." Mama Day calls him "an out-and-out bootlegger and con man" who sells "hoodoo bits of rags and sticks" and "watered-down moonshine" passed off as medicine (*Mama Day*, 51). Tucker's category is, however, a bit of an oversell of Buzzard's powers. Ruby, another conjure woman, uses her powers toward evil and is accused by the narrator of having committed two murders by poisoning.

Tucker says that Ruby's work against Cocoa is "straight conjure" and that there is nothing mysterious about her use of nightshade and snakeroot. She admits, however, that "other illnesses—the welts, Cocoa's 'hallucinations' which are not quite that, the strange appearances of the worms—are common symptoms of conjure told many times in many places yet never quite believed. Nor are they explained away by Naylor, who allows some of the more mysterious events to coexist with the more 'natural' ones in this text of many stories."[25]

In at least one instance, Mama Day's powers are clearly related to her common sense and her highly skilled use of natural remedies.[26] Summoned to Carmen Rae's sick baby, Mama Day sees what she expected: "the flushed face, his little chest heaving as the air whistles through his clogged throat" (*Mama Day*, 192). Too sick to cry, the baby whimpers, and Mama Day sets to work. She is furious, however, with the baby's mother, whose house is filthy.

> She scrapes off the caked grease from inside the pots, and while boiling them down in two changes of water, she scalds the countertops before opening her canvas pouch and laying her dried herbs out on them. She don't use much: all together it's only a teaspoon of senna pods, coltsfoot, horehound, white cherry bark, and black cohosh set to steep into the third change of water. She weighs them out by touch—some the roots, some the leaves, some the whole plant. [*Mama Day*, 193]

Using a charcoal brazier as a vaporizer with horehound leaves, carefully measured, since "the baby's misery calls for more, his body weight for less" (*Mama Day*, 193), Mama Day cradles the baby in her arms throughout the night, giving him tablespoons of the mixture and awaits his healing, which comes about by morning. There is nothing mysterious about this treatment; the description of it allows readers to see into Mama Day's expertise. She becomes a fully believable character in this novel, and much as Dr. Smithfield cannot write her off, neither can readers.

More complicated are Mama Day's dealings with Bernice, a high-strung young woman desperate to become pregnant who approaches Mama Day for help. Mama Day orders her to stay away from fertility drugs or to go see Dr. Smithfield, who himself "don't believe in them things." She gives Bernice star grass and raspberry teas and "a little something for [her] nerves" (*Mama Day*, 43), knowing from her reading of a chicken egg that the time for Bernice to get pregnant has not yet come. Miranda fails to read Bernice's desperation correctly, however, and later is summoned by her terrified husband, Ambush. She finds Bernice with a high fever and in excruciating pain from the perganol she has stolen from the pharmacy where she works. Mama Day smells the fever, "a dry burning," and proceeds to diagnose her:

> With the back of her hand, Miranda feels Bernice's forehead and the side of her neck. She lifts Bernice's wrist and feels for the rhythm of the blood while pressing her ear against her chest. Then she pulls back her eyelids and makes her roll her eyes around. . . .
>
> "Now, where is the pain, Bernice?"
>
> "In my stomach."
>
> "You sure it's your stomach?" She turns Bernice on her back and makes her fold her hands gently on her belly. "Close your eyes and try to concentrate on the pain. Is it coming from your stomach for true?" . . .
>
> "No, Mama Day, it's my sides." Bernice winces.
>
> Miranda nods. "And what kind of pain is it, Bernice?"
>
> "It hurts."
>
> "I know it hurts, honey, but is it like little needles all in one spot or does it kinda radiate out and down?"
>
> "It's like it's happening in my stomach and side all at one time." [*Mama Day*, 73]

Sounding a bit like the questions from a Melzack pain question-naire,[27] Mama Day's methods are subtle and precise. Mama Day carefully palpates Bernice's stomach and sides. She confirms that Bernice is not pregnant and is pretty certain that the fever will not be broken "from the outside." To make sure, she sniffs Bernice's urine and knows that there is "pus" in her "upper parts." She also performs an internal exam:

> Miranda slides her fingers up into Bernice real gentle. Them wrinkled fingers had gone that way so many times for so many different reasons. A path she knew so well that the slightest change of moisture, the amount of give along the walls, or the scent left on her hands could fix a woman's cycle within less than a day of what was happen-ing with the moon. . . . When she moves her . . . hand a fraction to the side and bears down a bit harder, a spot the size of a dime sends off blazing heat. Bernice cries out and tenses her legs. [*Mama Day*, 75–76]

Mama Day diagnoses an infected ovary and blocked tubes, thus explaining why Bernice has missed her period and still is not preg-nant. She sends Ambush for Brian Smithfield, the physician across the bridge, since she is dealing with chemicals and knows well her own limits. Before Smithfield comes, however, Miranda makes a pain medication for Bernice:

> Miranda washes off the choke-cherry bark and then cuts a piece about the size of the last joint on her little finger. She has to be careful with this stuff—awful careful. It could kill as easy as cure. And there weren't no time to dry it out and make a syrup. She props Bernice up in her arms and first makes her suck on a piece of peppermint candy. . . . When Bernice has worked up a good spit, Miranda takes the candy from her. "Now, Bernice, I want you to put this here piece of bark in your mouth and chew good. I'm warning

you that it's bitter, but try not to gag. Keep moving it
around in there, 'cause if it stay in one spot it's gonna burn
the lining of your mouth." [*Mama Day*, 82]

Miranda alternates the candy with the bark until "Bernice's body
start[s] to relax [and] her breath [comes] in a little deeper" (*Mama
Day*, 82). When the doctor arrives, he confirms Mama Day's diagnosis and treatment.

The working relationship between Mama Day and Smithfield is
worth examining. The shared respect between the two and their
ability (and desire) to work together is a useful model for modern
medicine.

> Each knew their limitations and where to draw the
> line. . . . He had a measure of respect for the way things
> was done here. It just saved him a lot of aggravation. No
> point in prescribing treatment for gout, bone inflamma-
> tion, diabetes, or even heart trouble when the person's
> going straight to Miranda after seeing him for her yea or
> nay. And if it was nay, she'd send 'em right back to him
> with a list of reasons. Better to ask straight out how she
> been treating 'em and work around that. Although it hurt
> his pride at times, he'd admit inside that it was usually no
> different than what he had to say himself—just plainer
> words and a slower cure than them concentrated drugs.
> And unless there was just no other choice, she'd never cut
> on nobody. Only twice in recollection, she'd picked up a
> knife. [*Mama Day*, 84]

Miranda operated on a water moccasin bite and performed an emergency cesarean section ("them stitches on Reema's stomach was neat
as a pin and she never set up a fever"). This is not an idealized
relationship, however. Smithfield knows that if he competes with
Mama Day, his life will be complicated, aggravated. The key to Smithfield's wisdom, however, is his ability to know his own limits and

suspend his judgment about what he simply cannot understand: "Being an outsider, he couldn't be expected to believe the other things Miranda could do. But being a good doctor, he knew another one when he saw her" (*Mama Day*, 84). Smithfield stays connected to a community not his own through Mama Day and his patients and thus is able to serve them better.

Mama Day continues to work with Bernice in her desperate quest to become pregnant. Sounding much like Minnie Ransom in *The Salt Eaters* ("You sure, sweetheart, you want to be well?"), Mama Day says to Bernice, "I can help you if you willing to work with me as hard as you worked on that [baby's] room" (*Mama Day*, 87). Treating her with good common sense, she gives Bernice painted pumpkin seeds, some black and some gold. The black seeds are for carrying negative energy into the ground; the gold, to "let the life blood flow out of you into this seed" whenever her monthly period comes (*Mama Day*, 97). In addition, Mama Day has Bernice cooking from scratch, cleaning, exercising, and using her creative energies in positive ways, rather than worrying over becoming pregnant. A few months later at the new moon, Mama Day takes Bernice out to the "other place," the home in which Miranda and her sister Abigail grew up, the site of much pain and sadness (but also where Sapphira Wade performed her conjure). Mama Day performs a fertility ritual with Bernice that appears full of strange magic, but which the narrator claims was perfectly natural: "She wasn't changing the natural course of nothing, she couldn't if she tried. Just using what's there. And couldn't be nothing wrong in helping Bernice to believe that there's something more than there is" (*Mama Day*, 139). For this ritual, Mama Day brings a laying hen with her and waits for Bernice to arrive once the moon has risen. When she does, Mama Day breaks an egg that the hen lays and Bernice eats it raw. Inside the house, the hen lays another egg directly into Bernice's vagina, with help from Mama Day's fingers.

> Her shoulders, sides, and stomach made into something
> more liquid than water, her breasts and hips flowing up

against the pull of the earth. She ain't flesh, she's a center
between the thighs spreading wide to take in . . . the touch
of feathers. . . . Ancient fingers keeping each in line. The
uncountable, the unthinkable, is one opening. Pulsing and
alive—wet—the egg moves from one space to the other. A
rhythm older than woman draws it in and holds it tight.
[*Mama Day*, 140]

Later, Bernice becomes pregnant. Would she have become pregnant
without this mysterious ritual? Was it a matter of mind over body?
Whose story counts? After Bernice has the baby, she repudiates her
relationship with Mama Day, perhaps ashamed of her dependence on
her, perhaps afraid that the work with Mama Day was more effectual
than her own attempts with medical technology (the perganol). And
although Mama Day insists that her methods are simply "natural,"
she later blames herself for "meddling" with nature when Bernice's
baby dies.

Ruby is also creative and resourceful, but she uses her knowledge
for evil. Obsessively jealous, Ruby had seduced her current husband,
Junior Lee, from his wife after working roots on him. Ruby's powers
are not insignificant; Junior Lee is functionally her slave. People are
afraid of Ruby's rootwork; Miranda, who states, "The mind is everything," insists to Junior Lee's former wife that it is futile to try to win
him back. The narrator insists that it is not magic that empowers
Miranda or Ruby, but their understanding of the mind's power and
how they use it and to what purpose. How is it, then, that Ruby is
able to make Cocoa so desperately and grotesquely ill? And what is
the explanation for Mama Day's powers of seeing and healing?

All of the interpretative difficulties are thrown into bold relief
when Cocoa falls ill as the result of Ruby's jealousy and rootworking
spells, and Cocoa's husband, George, reacts with utter disbelief, frantic to get Cocoa a "real" doctor to cure her horrible malady. George,
who grew up in an orphanage under the care of a woman who was
nothing if not a realist, has trouble with the world of Willow Springs
anyway, and he struggles to respect and believe in the way of life that

to him seems unnecessarily closed off from the wonders of modern technology. Mrs. Jackson, George's caretaker at the Wallace P. Andrews Shelter for Boys, repeatedly enjoined the boys to "keep it in the now, fellas. . . . Only the present has potential, *sir*" (*Mama Day*, 22–23; emphasis in original). George's admiration for Mrs. Jackson rests in the fact that the boys who left her care did not end up being "burden[s] on the state. . . . I don't know of anyone who became a drug addict, petty thief, or a derelict. I guess it's because you grew up with absolutely no illusions about yourself or the world" (*Mama Day*, 26). George has a heart condition and has grown up with no illusions about his body, either. Fiercely committed to healthy diet and exercise, George respects Mama Day's attention to health as well. But once Cocoa becomes deathly ill, George's respect turns to fear.

It is small wonder that George cannot believe that Cocoa's illness is what it is. As storm clouds gather, Ruby offers to fix Cocoa's hair in cornrows. Using a special white twine and digging the comb in "just short of hurting" (*Mama Day*, 246), Ruby massages a solution from an assortment of jars into her scalp. Once finished, Ruby, smiling, watches Cocoa walk toward home and "brushes a few strands from her lap into her hand and puts them in her pocket" (*Mama Day*, 247). A few hours later Cocoa begins to have viral symptoms, fever, headache, lassitude, and extreme fatigue, as though her "motions were all underwater and the sleep was quickly overtaking [her]" (*Mama Day*, 254). George is confused and panicky and wants to get her to a doctor immediately, "or at least call one about your symptoms, so we'd know what to do" (*Mama Day*, 260). George sees Cocoa's "glassy look" and diagnoses her with "brain fever," but Miranda has seen the red splotches and sniffed at the scalp and knows immediately it is nightshade. Ruby has anticipated this, hoping that Miranda would think that was all she had done. "Miranda lifts [the braids] up in her hand, watching the little red welts that are beginning on her neck and spreading down to her shoulders. She runs her fingertips over one and it causes her to shiver. She ain't really understood what it meant till now—that killing's too good for somebody." When she cuts Cocoa's braids close to the head, they fall "curled up like worms," and when the white strings come out of the braids, they look "even more like worms. Maggots, really. She's gotta force herself to go on until each plait is loosened" (*Mama Day*, 264). Using charcoal paste to draw what poison she can from Cocoa's scalp, she realizes that "the rest was just about out of her hands" (*Mama Day*, 265). When Abigail asks Miranda how bad it is, Miranda responds with a question, "How bad is hate, Abigail? How strong is hate?" (*Mama Day*, 267).

Mama Day vents her rage at Ruby's treachery, throwing silver powder into Ruby's yard: "She strikes the house in the back. Powder. She strikes it on the left. Powder. She brings the cane over her head and strikes it so hard against the front door, the window panes rattle," and she leaves a "circle of silvery powder" around Ruby's house. Lightning strikes twice, and the house explodes with Ruby in it. George, puzzled at the two strikes in the same place, recognizes the phenomenon only in terms of the unlikely event that someone had undertaken a "scientific enterprise" and simply cannot imagine the reality even when he names it: "Unless, of course, in a scientific experiment someone purposely electrifies the ground with materials that hold both negative and positive charges to increase the potential of having a target hit" (*Mama Day*, 274). George's fealty to technology and modern science renders him oblivious to Mama Day's power and knowledge.

In fact, George seems almost to prefer ignorance to insight as the situation worsens. Mama Day tells him, "I can tell you the truth, which you won't believe, or I can invent a lie, which you would. Which would you rather have?" (*Mama Day*, 266). Furious with her, he refuses to answer. Meanwhile, Cocoa's red welts are spreading all over her body, and she begins having hallucinations, thinking it is a phenomenon of the virus with which she believes she is infected. "The flesh from both cheeks was now hanging in strings under my ears, and moving my head caused them to wiggle like hooked worms." After washing her face, Cocoa sees that "my eyes, lips, chin, forehead, and ears had been smeared everywhere, mashed in and wrinkled, with some gouged places still holding the imprints from

my fingers and the terrycloth" (*Mama Day*, 276). Cocoa's grandmother, Abigail, is not surprised when she hears her scream, and she
covers all the mirrors in the house with cloth, knowing the power of
nightshade—but also that the nightshade is but a beginning of Ruby's
malevolent work. Abigail's quiet care and her constant singing of
hymns does not hide her sure knowledge of the evil visited on Cocoa
and her deep fear for her granddaughter's life.

Cocoa's condition worsens as Miranda spends time at the "other
place," attempting to learn from her ancestors and, indeed, dreams of
her mother, whose suicide Miranda recalls with a great deal of pain.
She pieces together the ragged years that followed her mother's death
and comes to the understanding that somehow she and George
would be "the bridge for Baby Girl to walk over" (*Mama Day*, 285).
Meanwhile, Cocoa begins to feel the welts

> itching as they curled and stretched themselves, multiply-
> ing as they burrowed deeper into [her] flesh. . . . I'm trying
> to remember when I felt that I was slipping beyond help. It
> wasn't with the realization that they were spreading so
> rapidly because they were actually feeding on me, the pu-
> trid odor of decaying matter that I could taste on my
> tongue and smell with every breath I took. Or my urine
> coming thick and brown with little flecks of the lining from
> my bladder left on the toilet tissue. [*Mama Day*, 287]

The maggots function much like hatred as they infest Cocoa's body
and gnaw at it from the inside out, "like the scraping of rough cloth,
inside of me" (*Mama Day*, 290). Ruby has displaced her hatred into
Cocoa's body, and it eats Cocoa rather than herself.

The storm that brought the lightning to Ruby also washes out the
bridge to the mainland, and there is no way to bring a doctor over to
tend Cocoa. Rather than seeing that he must *become* the bridge,
George is nearly hysterical in his frustration and works feverishly
with the other men to rebuild it. He is determined to get across the
water, even if by rowboat, although he cannot swim. George con-

tinues to think that Cocoa's illness is something that medical technology can cure, but Miranda attempts to convince him otherwise: "You see, she done bound more than her flesh up with you. And since she's suffering from something more than the flesh, I can't do a thing without you" (*Mama Day*, 294). Only when George sees for himself that the "worms" he believes Cocoa is hallucinating are, indeed, real does he become motivated to listen to Mama Day. When Cocoa showers, she sees the water coming thick out of the nozzle and that "there was a difference in the weight of the long watery beads clinging to my flesh. Before I knew it, they were pouring down over me and crawling into every opening of my body— some even pushing their way in through the corners of my lips" (*Mama Day*, 297). George sees in Cocoa "the hollow eyes of a lunatic" and takes her to bed to comfort her, making love and telling her that it was "only water" in the shower. After they have sex, however, he discovers a piece of worm on his penis. "I smashed it between my fingers. It left a yellowish smear with the odor of rotting garbage" (*Mama Day*, 298). Stunned by the inexplicable, George becomes willing to follow Mama Day's instructions, although reluctantly and with no little skepticism, as she tells him to go to the chicken coop and bring her what he finds at the bottom of the hen's nest. When he panics and fights the rooster, he dies of a heart attack, but in his willingness to listen to Mama Day and help Cocoa, he has indeed become the bridge over which she will be able to walk toward health.[28]

Hardly the stuff of an urban emergency room or medical clinic, the illnesses and traumas of Willow Springs nevertheless hold within them the tensions implicit in a narrative approach to ethics: Whom should one trust? Whose story holds weight? Why? What is going on? And, of course, What to do? While *Mama Day* is clearly not a primer for understanding or even appreciating "alternative" medicine, it does challenge readers to think about the ways stories weave themselves together and how, in the weaving, truth is apprehended bit by bit. It challenges readers not to fall into the trap of the anthropologist who could not even figure out the right questions to ask but, instead, to listen carefully and to listen to highly unlikely sources and improbable voices that make up such a community as Willow Springs (or the streets of Watts or West Chicago or New York). It is a novel that resists medical colonization in its opaqueness, but it also simultaneously invites medicine to reconsider its relationship with the communities of people it serves and its assumptions about hierarchies of knowing. For in Naylor's novel, Mama Day's ways of knowing are equal, if not superior, to Dr. Smithfield's, and he, being no fool, understands and makes good use of her expertise.

Told in a fashion that Sandra Cisneros says resembles a rowdy *tele-novela*, Ana Castillo's So *Far from God*, less known and less attended to than *Mama Day*, similarly confounds readers' needs for explanation and truth. It also levels a critique at technological medicine's misuses and its ineffectiveness in healing certain kinds of ailments. Castillo explains a tendency that I believe informs her literary method.

> A growing trend among those of us who are pursuing non-traditional lifestyles is to return to long lost and non-Western ways in search of new direction for our lives; we have unearthed the ways of our Mexic Amerindian ancestors preserved by our mestizo elders, most often, women, in the form of curanderismo. . . . The Arabic medical practice of utilizing herbal cures was readapted in the Americas with plants found on these continents and combined with Native American healing knowledge, which, in addition to herbal medicine, also has included baths, setting bones, and other remedies.[29]

For Castillo, the reclamation of such practices is a matter of survival as well as celebration. She notes that "some feminist-activists in the mental health services are using these methods with their Latino/a clientele, which seems to respond more effectively to this treatment than to the alien mental health practices of the white establishment."[30] It is out of Castillo's commitment to bringing denigrated or marginalized beliefs and practices to the center that *So Far from God* emerges.

Drawing on Chicano culture and traditional beliefs about healing and illness, the novel lays out the lives of a matriarchal family. The insightful and at times hilarious narrator describes Sofi, the (wise) mother, as one who "single-handedly ran the Carne Buena Carnecería she inherited from her parents. She raised most of the livestock that she herself . . . butchered for the store, managed all its finances, and ran the house on her own to boot" (*So Far*, 28). She is but one among a number of strong women in the novel who embrace nontraditional healing. The novel begins with a disaster and a *milagro* when Sofi's three-year-old baby suffers a violent seizure (so violent that the animals are disturbed, "kicking and crying and running back and forth with their ears back and fur standing on end" [*So Far*, 19]). After her eyes have rolled up into her head, she appears dead, a diagnosis confirmed by the young doctor at the county clinic. During the funeral mass a few days later, however, the baby revives: "The [coffin] lid had pushed all the way open and the little girl inside sat up, just as sweetly as if she had woken from a nap, rubbing her eyes and yawning" (*So Far*, 22). This would be miracle enough, but the child flies to the church roof and warns the people not to touch her, thus marking her lifelong phobia of people ("She claimed that all humans bore an odor akin to that which she had smelled in the places she had passed through when she was dead" [*So Far*, 23]). The Albuquerque hospital diagnoses her with probable epilepsy, but as the understated narrator adds, "there was much left unexplained." The narrator recalls how the oddball Franky el Penetente, a Vietnam veteran and carver of sacred santos, had experienced the event years earlier:

> Despite what anyone wanted to say or not about the elusive youngest daughter, she could not be of this world, having returned from the dead before a hundred witnesses. . . . And when little Franky . . . [had seen] the child

fly up to the church roof, man! What he wouldn't have
given to know the secret of that trick! To the boy it was a
trick, the way all children view the magical, which to them
falls within the realm of possibility. [*So Far*, 192]

The rational sister, Fe, however, has always suspected that *El Milagro*,
La Loca's resurrection, never happened, and furthermore, she "did
not feel compassion for La Loca . . . but simply disappointment and
disgust for her sister's obvious 'mental illness,' the fact that her
mother had encouraged it with her own superstitions, and finally,
fear that it was, like her own Indian flat butt, hereditary, despite
everyone's protest to the contrary" (*So Far*, 29). The truth of the
event thus remains contested for years after its occurrence.[31]

The community gives the child the name La Loca Santa, but later
the "Santa" is dropped and she becomes known as La Loca to all,
including her family.[32] La Loca continues to avoid human contact.
"Only her mother and the animals [are] ever unconditionally allowed
to touch her. But without exception, healing her sisters from the
traumas and injustices they were dealt by society—a society she
herself never experienced firsthand—was never questioned" (*So
Far*, 27).

Of the sisters, there is Esperanza (hope) who got her B.A. in
Chicano studies at the university, has "spunk," and becomes a news
broadcaster at a local TV station. Her sister Fe (faith), despises Esperanza's "La Raza" politics and is overly eager to be a cookie-cutter
middle-class American woman. Fe, the voice of rationality—one with
whom middle-class, educated readers might at first identify or whom
they might at least trust, but for the narrator's tone—has a job at the
bank and a hard-working fiancé. After he jilts her, Fe temporarily
loses her mind, screaming for months, disrupting the household, and
driving the family nearly crazy with the incessant noise. What finally
quiets Fe is her sister Caridad's miraculous cure.

Caridad (charity), the beautiful sister, had attended college for a
year and married Memo, also for a year, after getting pregnant, di-
vorced, and "all in all . . . [having] had three abortions. . . . La Loca had

performed each one. . . . It would have been a terrible thing to let anyone find out that La Loca had 'cured' her sister of her pregnancy, a cause for excommunication for both, not to mention that someone would have surely had La Loca arrested. A crime against man if not a sin against God" (*So Far*, 26– 27). Caridad's fondness for liquor with beer chasers and sexual promiscuity lands her in serious trouble when she is brought home one night "a nightmare incarnated . . . as mangled as a stray cat" (*So Far*, 32–33). (Months later the *curandera* Doña Felicia will discern that her attacker had been "pure force" and "had no shape and was darker than the dark night" [*So Far*, 77]). "There was too much blood to see at the time, but after Caridad had been taken by ambulance to the hospital, treated and saved (just barely), Sofi was told that her daughter's nipples had been bitten off. She had also been scourged with something, branded like cattle. Worst of all, a tracheotomy was performed because she had also been stabbed in the throat" (*So Far*, 33). After three months in the hospital, "what was left" of Caridad comes home to the care of her family (and Fe's continual screaming). Shortly thereafter, right after one of La Loca's infrequent seizures, Caridad (or what Sofi thinks is a vision of her) emerges from the bedroom, "whole and once again beautiful . . . in what . . . appeared to be Fe's wedding gown. . . . Sofi stepped back when she saw, not what had been left of her daughter, half repaired by modern medical technology, tubes through her throat, bandages over skin that was gone, surgery piecing together flesh that was once her daughter's breasts, but Caridad as she was before. . . . Caridad was whole" (*So Far*, 37–38). The juxtaposition of the Caridad who returns from the hospital's ministrations and the Caridad of the miracle is a striking and pointed reference to the "half" repair modern technology could give her. Indeed, the narrator makes her opinion of technological medicine clear as she witnesses Caridad's whole and beautifully restored body. At the same time, and just as miraculously, Fe stops screaming and rocks her sister, "stroking her forehead, humming softly to her" (*So Far*, 38).

After Caridad's "Holy Restoration," as her mother calls it, she goes to live in a trailer with her horse, Corazón. Her landlady is the well-known *curandera* Doña Felicia, who looks "like she was at least ninety years old" but tells stories of fighting in the Mexican Civil War, and so must have been older. Despite her age, Doña Felicia embroiders without glasses, watches her favorite *telenovelas* on Spanish cable TV (in between her patients), and is always "ready with a pot of coffee and plate of beans to make you feel right at home" (*So Far*, 44). She tells Caridad that she set bones and removed bullets during the *Revolución* ("and more importantly, I gave them courage!" [*So Far*, 55]).

Healed, Caridad returns to work at the hospital (to "change starched linen, clean out bedpans, help make patients comfortable, fluff up their pillows, and get hold of doctors to prescribe heavier doses of medication when they couldn't sleep because of so much pain and misery" [*So Far*, 50– 51]). She repudiates her old ways, having quit drinking and "dating," but there is more. Caridad begins to discover that she herself is a healer. In fact, when she begins going into trance states (some of which last days at a time) and, like Loca, foretells the future from time to time,[33] Doña Felicia begins to suspect that Caridad has the gift of healing. By putting Caridad in a hospital and then taking her out when she discovers her gift, Castillo raises a question about the kinds of healers institutional medicine can tolerate. She also critiques the hospital by making it a place inhospitable to Caridad's healing gifts.

Doña Felicia reverses medical hierarchies as she tells Caridad she is a more important healer than doctors and nurses because Caridad knows the difference between foresight and prevention, "two important aspects of the laws of the universe," and that this is "an indication of a true healer" (*So Far*, 54–55). Doña Felicia tells Caridad that she is

> meant to help people a lot more than just wiping their be-
> hinds as they make you do in the hospital. . . . You are des-
> tined to help people as even those trained doctors and
> nurses down there can't do. Look what you did for your-
> self! All they did at the hospital was patch you up and send

you home, more dead than alive. It was with the help of
God, heaven knows how He watches over that house
where you come from. . . . But *you* healed yourself by pure
will. And yes, I will show you all I know. It will be my pleasure and it is el Señor's wish. [*So Far*, 55–56]

After a preparatory fourteen-day sleep, Caridad begins her apprenticeship by listening to Doña Felicia, who sets her own life in context,
knowing that healing is, in part, about understanding a lifetime of
stories. She recounts that she lost her mother to malnourishment and
untreated disease and that she became, as a result, "suspicious of the
religion that did not help the destitute all around her despite their
devotion." After her first husband died in Zapata's army, she developed a faith that was "based not on an institution but on the bits and
pieces of the souls and knowledge of the wise teachers that she met
along the way" (*So Far*, 60). Very much in keeping with the tradition
of *curandismo*, Doña Felicia tells Caridad, "Nothing you attempt to do
with regards to healing will work without first placing your faith
completely in God" (*So Far*, 59).[34]

As she tells her story to Caridad, Doña Felicia instructs her in the
art of listening. In fact, diagnosis, Felicia tells Caridad, is so much a
matter of listening ("Could Caridad even be said to know how to
listen at all, much less listen properly so as to not misdiagnose an
illness? A curandera not only had the health of her patient in her own
hands but the spirit as well" [*So Far*, 62]). Moreover, a *curandera*
needed "an abundant heart" and "resiliency" (*So Far*, 77). In addition, Caridad must learn discernment, how to determine which
symptoms "were based on physical ailments . . . spiritual factors, and
which were 'psychological'—and therefore to be treated solely with
generous doses of compassion." As Mama Day knows, Doña Felicia
tells Caridad, "Everything we need for healing is found in our natural
surroundings" (*So Far*, 62). The most common ailments, she tells her,
are *empacho* and *bilis, mal de ojo, caida de mollera, susto,* and *aigre.*
"These illnesses could be a result of physical causes or . . . the result
of someone's bad intentions," since "envy was a formidable force . . .

which could cause a victim to suffer the worst pain imaginable, even death!" (*So Far*, 63).[35] Doña Felicia underscores the wisdom of contextualizing a patient's illness by showing how understanding a patient's lifeworld is essential to diagnosis and healing and is not simply a nicety of the healer-patient relationship. Her remedies include, for example, massage for *empacho*, but she also acknowledges that such a malady derives frequently from such things as "a sorrow too great to contain any longer, anxiety over not having work to support one's family, or misery caused by an unfaithful lover." The purpose of a cleansing is, she says, "to restore peace of mind to the individual, to give him a clear head so that he will know what practical things he must do to improve his lot" (*So Far*, 69). The connection, for Doña Felicia, between body and spirit is so seamless as to be nearly invisible to her. It is simply a given.

Caridad's apprenticeship proceeds uneventfully until she disappears for a year, stunned by her passion for a nameless woman she had encountered on a pilgrimage to Chimayo. Once she is discovered living in a cave as an ascetic, Caridad finds herself a reluctant but sensational cult figure with hundreds of followers making pilgrimages to *her*. Mostly oblivious to the activity around her, Caridad returns home and begins to interpret dreams, with Doña Felicia's help. Somewhat like Minnie Ransom of *The Salt Eaters*, Caridad "communicate[s] with spirit guides as a way of communicating messages to clients" (*So Far*, 119), and Franky el Penetente (who is hopelessly in love with her) sees a glow emanating from Caridad's body. Despite the narrator's wry observation that Franky habitually thought "he was making sagacious connections when he wasn't even plugged in" (*So Far*, 204), Franky declares that this vision "was not delirium" but was instead a truth, "nothing short of a blessing, an unmerited reward for the physical suffering he was imposing on himself as penance" (*So Far*, 192). The question of interpretation continues as Caridad and her by-now-found love, Esmeralda, jump off the mesa together: "Just the spirit deity Tsichtinako calling loudly with a voice like wind, guiding the two women back, not out toward the sun's rays or up to the clouds but down, deep within the soft, moist dark earth where Esmeralda and Caridad would be safe and live forever" (*So Far*, 211). The bodies are never found. What is going on? The narrator gives us her version: the two women have found their place in the earth and are alive, eternally safe together.

Interpretation is challenged once again through La Loca. By now Fe is dead, Esperanza's murder as a journalist in the Persian Gulf has been confirmed (and she returns as a spirit from time to time), and Caridad is living somewhere in the earth's embrace with Esmeralda. La Loca begins to notice that her jeans are getting baggier, and Sofi calls the family doctor. Dr. Tolentino, a graduate of Northwestern University Medical School ("in the coldest city in the world" [*So Far*, 227]), is "one of those old-fashioned general-family-practice-type doctors," the description of which the narrator uses to vent her spleen at hospitals and modern medicine once again. She continues: "The kind [of doctor] people only find in rural areas nowadays, and not always there no more, really, since women in labor in such places can be helicoptered to hospitals during snowstorms, and very sick people don't die peacefully at home no more but are forced to a strange bed in a hospital, days and even weeks before their time" (*So Far*, 223). Tolentino diagnoses HIV infection, and Sofi is sure of only two things: "that there was no known cure for this frightening epidemic and . . . there was no way that Loca could have gotten it" (*So Far*, 226). Indeed, the etiology of her HIV is perplexing, given Loca's abhorrence of human contact.

Dr. Tolentino and his wife, the daughter of a missionary in Tome from years earlier, offer to provide a *tratimento* to Loca, explaining to Sofi that since "we are now in the age of the Spirit," they would begin the treatment by praying together. Tolentino rubs holy oil on Loca's stomach, asking her to breathe deeply when there is a "popping sound."

> La Mrs. Doctor had soaked a handful of cotton balls with holy oil and squeezed them over Loca's tummy. Doctor Tolentino dripped a cotton ball in a pan of warm water and as he dripped the water on Loca's stomach with his right

> hand, his left hand made an opening through her flesh and
> disappeared right up to the wrist inside her stomach. . . .
> [Loca saw] the doctor's hand disappear into her body. She
> felt no pain, though she did find it hard to breathe deeply,
> as the doctor was telling her to do while the right hand also
> went inside her stomach, the opening maintained by the
> left one. In a few seconds he pulled out his right hand hold-
> ing a bloody coagulation which he held up for Loca's ap-
> praisal, explaining that it was a blood clot and then
> dropping it into the bowl of water his wife held out for
> him. [*So Far*, 228]

He enters her twice more, using the "material" hand to maintain the
opening and the "spirit" hand to seek the problems. When the doctor
finally removes his hand, there is only a "slender line of blood" as a
sign that surgery had been performed.[36] Sofi, meanwhile, convinces
herself—for the moment— that she has seen "nothing more than a
hallucination." Tolentino has absolute faith in his methods, but he
explains to Sofi and Loca that "although sometimes a disease could
be stopped, death ultimately could not be" (*So Far*, 229). Tolentino
and Doña Felicia alternate visits, but they all know (including Loca)
that "no cure was forthcoming." Predictably, La Loca wants nothing
to do with institutionalized medicine: "The atrocities that [she] saw
Fe suffer in her last days on the Acme International Medical Group
Plan were enough to keep her far away from anyone wearing anything that even looked like a smock as long as she lived" (*So Far*,
230). In La Loca's eventual death, the issues of uncertainty (Did the
psychic surgery really happen? How did Loca, who despised human
contact, get AIDS? Who was the mysterious ghostly woman with
whom she regularly conversed at the creek? Was it the mythical La
Llorona? Who was the blue woman she saw as she died?) and the
sociopolitical roots of disease come together.

The only events not open to interpretation are those surrounding
Fe's illness and death. Significantly, Fe is the only one of the dead
sisters who is truly and unequivocally dead. (Loca, like Esperanza,

makes appearances after her death.) In Fe's story, Castillo delivers her most strident critique of the American dream, the American military industry, modern biomedicine, and the politics of health. Much like the other authors in this study, Castillo connects Fe's illness clearly with unjust society and immoral politics. Fe's desire to obtain "the long-dreamed-of-automatic dishwasher, microwave, Cuisinart, and the VCR" keeps her obsessed with her work, ever vigilant to prove "what a good worker she was." After she is fired from her bank job because she has difficulty speaking clearly (as a result of the screaming), Fe takes a job at Acme International, a plant under contract to clean equipment for the weapons industry. Fe's job not only provides her with good raises but also gives her "nausea and headaches that increased in severity by the day." The nurse gives ibuprofen to the women at the plant, and Fe continues to "[take] on every gritty job available" (*So Far*, 178). She begins to worry when she discovers that several women have had miscarriages and/or hysterectomies since coming to Acme, but she continues working and accepts the unrelenting headaches that have become part of her daily routine.

Fe works with one chemical that glows in the dark and causes her to develop a "red ring around her nose and breath that smell[s] suspiciously of glue" (*So Far*, 181). She is also given what the plant managers call "ether" to clean machine parts in a closed room without ventilation or protective mask. She works with the chemical until it eats the gloves she is wearing and dissolves her fingernail polish and then the fingernails themselves. "Meanwhile," the narrator tells us, "the red ring around the nose, glue breath, big dried spots on her legs, and one constant fire drill going on in her head were doing nothing for her once-a-fairy-tale life with [her husband] Casey" (*So Far*, 185).

Predictably, Fe is diagnosed with cancer, "on the outside and all over the inside and there was no stopping it by then." (In addition, she is subpoenaed by the government for using the illegal substance provided to her to clean the equipment at work.) The medical treatment she receives is absolute "torture":

"First they went about removing the cancerous moles on her legs and arms and eventually, chest and back and then whole body, so that Fe's flesh almost at once was scarred all over. Having her whole body surgically scraped was agony enough, but then to add to this, the stress of the mysterious subpoena would cause these scars to swell from hives, and then Fe could not even walk" (*So Far*, 186–87). The hospital makes a "stupefying 'mistake' " when a catheter is fed through her collarbone and mistakenly goes up into her head, pouring chemotherapy into her brain rather than "down somewhere" in her body where it was supposed to go. "They thought they removed it when she left the hospital, but they hadn't. And until it was discovered because of an infection it caused and was finally pulled out, Fe went around feeling for seventy-one days and seventy-two nights like her brain wanted to pop out of her skull and nobody could figure out why, and they only kept insisting that it was all due to stress" (*So Far*, 187). And so Fe, "patched up and in perpetual pain," is released and waits at home to die, fully aware of what the chemical she had been working with has done to her ("it was . . . *heavier than air*" [*So Far*, 188; emphasis in original]). She despairs over the fact that at Acme, "everybody, meanwhile, was working in silence as usual" (*So Far*, 189).

Fe's story makes sense in light of Arthur Frank's observation that the "moral world" of physician and of patient frequently conflict. However, this is complicated in *So Far from God*. Frank, using the example of a community whose residents disproportionately suffered from cancer, states,

> The story told by residents of Tannerstown has to do with pollution, particularly from the factory that provides employment for many residents and fills the air with residues that most locals believe are toxic. The medical story has to do with people's high-fat diet, their smoking, and their alcohol consumption. [The] community members acknowledge their high cancer rates, but they interpellate themselves in a narrative of industrial exploitation. The

medical community sees the same cancer rates, cannot
make a determinative judgment about the effect of pollu-
tion, and claims "lifestyle" is the cause.[37]

Not only are Fe's narrative and the medical community's narrative in
conflict (Fe's pain is due to "stress"), but the novel also rejects any
claim the medical narrative might have. By drawing that narrative
into the text and exposing the self-interest of such a narrative—
complicity with the arms industry, failure to link Fe's personal troubles with social problems— the novel renders it impotent. *So Far from
God* carnivalizes the medical community, turning it upside down to
expose its soft underbelly.

Perhaps the circumstances of Fe's death, more than the others,
inspire Sofi to organize a Way of the Cross procession for the community that, much as do the tenets of liberation theology, establishes the
link between the suffering of people (and the unjust and immoral
causes of that suffering) and the suffering of Christ.

> No brother was elected to carry a life-size cross on his
> naked back. There was no "Mary" to meet her son. Instead,
> some, like Sofi, who held a picture of la Fe as a bride, car-
> ried photographs of their loved ones who died due to toxic
> exposure hung around the necks like scapulars; and at each
> station along their route, the crowd stopped and prayed
> and people spoke on the so many things that were killing
> their land and turning the people of those lands into an en-
> dangered species. [*So Far*, 241–42][38]

For example, at one station, "Jesus bore His cross and a man declared
that most of the Native and hispano families throughout the land
were living below poverty level." At another, "Jesus met his mother,
and three Navajo women talked about uranium contamination on the
reservation and the babies they gave birth to with brain damage and
cancer" (*So Far*, 242).[39]

In *So Far from God*, the only worship that makes any sense directly relates to a god interested in the reality and alleviation of suffering in this world. Health, injury, and illness are both mystery and fact of human existence *and* inextricably bound up with the evils of the world. Understanding whether Loca's resurrection was a medically explainable event or a miracle, or if Caridad really was miraculously cured, or if Tolentino actually conducted psychic surgery is all part of the mystery of living and dying—or more accurately, is the stuff of human attempts to understand and get it right. What is most important, for Castillo, is that suffering is *not* mysterious. It is something that is all too frequently rooted in human injustice and evil and, as such, is preventable, miracles or not.

Both *Mama Day* and *So Far from God* defer the question of making sense and, instead, push readers to ask questions and to hold possibilities up to the light, turning each carefully and thinking through various approaches to truth. These novels could be read almost as an apologia for narrative ethics. Attempts to find a unitary, linear, and mechanical explanation for all phenomena will be doomed to failure, they suggest. Instead, if the narrative itself is taken seriously, truths may emerge that enlighten patient, caregiver, and family alike. In addition, the respectful working relationship between Mama Day and Dr. Smithfield suggests a hopeful expansion of medicine's borders, a breaking-down of the hierarchies of power implicit in patient-physician relationships.

What happens, though, when contemporary biomedicine is faced with explanatory frameworks and healing practices that seem so counter to rational, believable explanations? Loudell Snow discusses the conflict that can occur when "superstitious" beliefs and practices are articulated in clinical settings:

> "But she seems to be an *intelligent* woman," one family
> practitioner kept repeating as he told me of the woman
> who had refused the surgical removal of uterine fibroids.
> What *he* viewed as a completely medical (and secular) sit-
> uation his patient took to be a tangible sign of divine dis-

pleasure. She understood the growths to be the deserved outcome of some unstated sinful behavior on her part and continued to firmly insist that God would heal her should it be His will; no scalpels necessary. . . . The strongly secular approach that is typical of biomedicine is in stark contrast to a health culture in which the most basic premises include aspects of the spiritual and supernatural.[40]

Such clashes in understanding and worldviews can be disastrous for both patient and physician alike. In her chronicle of what she calls the "collision of two cultures" between a Hmong family and their doctors, Anne Fadiman details the many ways the Lee family's interpretations of little Lia's epilepsy and the doctors' treatment of it led to devastating outcomes. Fadiman took the Lee's interpretations of Lia's illness to Arthur Kleinman for his "retroactive suggestions for her pediatricians." This is what he had to say to her:

First, get rid of the term, 'compliance.' It's a lousy term. It implies moral hegemony. You don't want a command from a general, you want a colloquy. Second, instead of looking at a model of coercion, look at a model of mediation. Go find a member of the Hmong community, or go find a medical anthropologist, who can help you negotiate. . . . Decide what's critical and be willing to compromise on everything else. Third, you need to understand that as powerful an influence as the culture of the Hmong patient and her family is on this case, the culture of biomedicine is equally powerful. If you can't see that your own culture has its own set of interests, emotions, and biases, how can you expect to deal successfully with someone else's culture?[41]

Kleinman calls for a different model, one that includes members of the community as consultants, or at least someone who can interpret the community to medicine (although *Mama Day*'s anthropologist provides a caution for this model). His advice to look at biomedicine as a culture of its own is in part what *Mama Day* and *So Far from God* do: they hold a mirror to medicine, illuminating its "interests, emotions, and biases" by representing not only the consequences but alternatives as well.

For what happens to the physician, functioning essentially as the practitioner (even among a team of such practitioners) who is isolated from the community from which many of her patients may come? She is left to use only what she has at her disposal: the tools of modern biomedicine. What if, instead, she was connected to healers within the community? Or even if she (or someone she knew or worked with) were able to consult and rally forces beyond hospital and clinic walls? Not only would the patient be better for this kind of collaboration, but the doctor herself would also be, for she would not be practicing in cultural and social isolation. Disease, trauma, death, and healing, the novels suggest, are ultimately beyond the ken of empirical biomedicine, but with careful listening and collaboration, medicine, unlike the failed anthropologist in *Mama Day*, might, with the help of the nonmedical community, understand, and learn something unexpected and healing—not just for the patient, but for itself as well.

Human Debris

Border Politics, Body Parts, and Anatomies of Medicine
in Leslie Marmon Silko's *Almanac of the Dead*

7

> I see *oposición e insurección*. I see the crack growing on the rock.
> I see the fine frenzy building. I see the heat of anger or
> rebellion or hope split open that rock, releasing *la Coatlicue*.
> —Gloria Anzaldúa, *Borderlands / La Frontera: The New Mestiza*

> What does it mean to say *I have survived*
> until you take the mirrors and turn them outward
> and read your own face in their outraged light?
> —Adrienne Rich, "Through Corralitos under Rolls of Cloud"

Much like Silko's *Ceremony*, *Almanac of the Dead* represents illness, but in strikingly different ways. *Ceremony* contextualizes individual illness, resistance, and healing in a manner that insists on the
integral connection between an individual sick body and a socially
sick world. In *Ceremony*, healing comes about as Tayo recognizes and
acknowledges that connection, as well as understanding the link
between his own illness and internalized as well as institutionalized
racism. In *Almanac*, however, the focus shifts from the social context
of individual illness to the context of institutionalized medicine itself. Medicine becomes, in a sense, the patient, struggling to function
within a diseased and infectious world. It is a context in which
murder, poverty, war, and the commodification of bodies and body
parts all undermine any semblance of moral order, a context in which
what an issue of *Daedalus* calls "social suffering" is the reality for all
but the exploitive and privileged few (and even those few are trapped
in their own self-made hells).[1] *Almanac* compels readers to look at
that context and to ask how it both profits and destroys medicine at
the same time.

Given the almost immediate outpouring of scholarly work on

Ceremony (1977), the early silence of literary scholars around *Almanac* (1991) was intriguing. (*Almanac* was met with nearly fifty reviews, however, ranging from ecstatic to grudgingly appreciative to hostile; while some reviewers criticized the novel for its violence and harshness, others hailed it as a masterpiece.)[2] Not until some six years after publication did more than a handful of critical articles on *Almanac* begin to appear in print.[3] *Almanac*'s difficult and harsh subject matter may, in part, explain the initial silence; there is little about which to feel good in Silko's sprawling tale. The novel critiques and challenges former and ongoing colonialism of the preceding 500 years in the Americas, and it marks a significant departure from Silko's previous work in both style and content. Told without the lyricism that characterizes much of *Ceremony*, *Almanac* presents brutal realities in unflinchingly stark language.

The novel is also structurally challenging. Sven Birkerts aptly comments that writing about *Almanac* is akin to "describing Rodin's 'The Gates of Hell' figure by figure."[4] *Almanac* is divided into seven parts: "The United States of America," "Mexico," "Africa," "Arizona," "The Americas," "The Fifth World," and "One World, Many Tribes." Each part contains one to eight "books"; most have geographic names ("The Border," "The North," etc.), but some have descriptive titles (such as "Reign of Death-Eye Dog," "The Foes," and "The Warriors"). Each book then contains short chapters (up to twenty-one), with such titles as "Abortion," "Suicide," "Shallow Graves," "Terrorist Bombs," "Vampire Capitalists," "Blood Madness," and "Spirit Macaws." With some seventy characters and a vast array of events spanning 500 years and several continents, *Almanac*'s plot is difficult to pin down. It is backgrounded in a textual field that represents, through its elaborate web, the cost of Western conquest, colonization, and oppression. Fashioned like the spider web structure Silko says is integral to Pueblo storytelling,[5] *Almanac*'s myriad characters and stories are intricately connected, although Silko states that she called the novel an almanac precisely because she had not planned for such connections.[6] What emerges in the writing represents an ancient circular Mayan almanac more than a Western almanac with its linear chronology, however.[7]

The voices and structures of the Mayan almanac tradition exist contrapuntally with the almost overwhelming almanac of the morally bankrupt living dead of the Euro-American twentieth century.[8]

Spatially, Tucson, Arizona, functions as a focal point in the novel, with much of the action radiating away from or toward the city. Arizona is about to go belly-up from the effects of a declining economy and devastating drought. As riots, uprisings, and civil wars plague Mexico, Central America, and South America, both U.S. and Mexican borders become clogged with those fleeing oppression and danger. Drawing on Native American and African beliefs, particularly Voodoo, Silko explains that she thinks of Tucson as a crossroads, since it was an important site on the pre-Columbian trade routes from New Mexico into Mexico, "a place of intense conflict between all the spirits, and all the forces."[9] As the prophecies have foretold, the people inexorably move northward, and while it may take 500 or 5,000 years, the indigenous will reclaim the diseased and corrupted land (and presumably become instruments of its healing).[10] The prophecy itself, inscribed on a map (drawn by Silko and reproduced on both endpapers), includes the reminder, "Sixty million Native Americans died between 1500 and 1600. . . . The defiance and resistance to things European continue unabated. Native Americans acknowledge no borders; they seek nothing less than the return of all tribal lands" (15),[11] and "when Europeans arrived, the Maya, Azteca, Inca cultures had already built great cities and vast networks of roads. Ancient prophecies foretold the arrival of Europeans in the Americas. The ancient prophecies also foretell the disappearance of all things European" (14).

Against this backdrop and into a complex milieu Silko inserts a host of unlikely characters that work—in one way or another—as part of the resistance. Among them are the twin sisters Lecha, a Demerol-addicted psychic who helps police locate the bodies of murder victims and has a lucrative profession as a talk show guest, and Zeta, who has made a fortune running drugs and guns across the North and South American borders with the help of Lecha's son and his sometime lover Paulie. There are also the twin brothers Tacho, who works both as chauffeur for the wealthy Menardo and as a spy for the indigenous resistance movement, and El Feo, who heads that movement in the far south of Mexico. Both brothers commune with spirit macaws for advice. Angelita, also known as La Escapía or "the Meat Hook,"[12] organizes the community for the violent overthrow of those in power while protecting the nonviolent projects of Tacho, El Feo, and their followers. Rambo Roy and Clinton (referred to as "the first Black Indian"), two homeless Green Beret Vietnam veterans in Tucson, organize the Army of the Homeless in an effort to retake "stolen" goods and land from the wealthy. In the north, Wilson Weasel Tail, a law school dropout and poet ("Only a bastard government / Occupies stolen land!" [714]), bills himself as "a Lakota healer and visionary" (716) and points out hopeful signs such as Euro-Americans having nervous breakdowns and psychotic episodes in "record numbers" (738). Another character, the Barefoot Hopi, "travel[s] the world to raise political and financial support for the return of the land to indigenous Americans" (616) and, himself an ex-convict, organizes incarcerated prisoners for a future uprising against the U.S. government. There is also Awa Gee, a computer genius who creates viruses and plans to disable computer systems nationally, along with the nation's electrical system ("Earth that was bare and empty . . . that had been seized and torn open, would be allowed to heal and to rest in the darkness after the lights were turned out" [683]). Many of these and other characters converge at the end of the novel at the (slightly wacky) International Holistic Healers Convention in Tucson, where "German root doctors" and "Celtic leech handlers" join "new-age spiritualists . . . [whites who] claimed to have been trained by 110-year-old Huichol Indians" (716) and the Green Vengeance eco-warriors.

Despite its comic aspects—and there are many, this hauntingly realistic novel describes a malaise that is devastating.[13] Alcohol and cocaine are the mainstay of the wealthy; sex is brutal and used as a tool for manipulation or base self-gratification (as in the example of Judge Arne and his "beloved bassett hounds" [655]); in Mexico City "trash cans are stuffed with newborns" (47); and the heads of the U.S.

ambassador to Mexico and his chief aide float in plastic shopping bags in the gardens of Xochimilco (164). But most horrible in this narrative are the forces for evil and the nightmare of the contemporary social contract in the Americas. Those who can afford to—many of the characters in *Almanac*—have gone mad with technological idolatry and avarice. Indeed, the lure of the infinite possibilities promised by technology is coupled with a widespread disregard for all human life that does not directly serve the interests of the wealthy. Together these forces create an atmosphere of social approbation for the manipulation of science and medicine by and for the most wealthy and powerful members of society. *Almanac* addresses complex medical and ethical issues in its focus on (among other things) the traffic in human organs, a laboratory where genetic manipulation and in vitro fertilization are placed in the service of creating a pure-blooded master race, and a "deep ecology" movement that recruits eco-warriors from the ranks of terminally ill AIDS patients (also hopeless in the face of a mostly indifferent government) to become human bombs ("Go out while you're still feeling good and *looking* good! / Avenge gay genocide by the U.S. government! / Die to save the earth. / Mold long underwear out of plastic explosives and stroll past the U.S. Supreme Court building while the justices are hearing arguments" [730]).[14]

Arnold Krupat writes that "contemporary Native American literatures tend to derive from an ecosystemic, nonanthropocentric perspective on the world" that is essential to human survival.[15] In *Almanac*, Silko creates a society that has, to put it mildly, failed to develop such a perspective. As Katherine Callen King says, "At the core of *Almanac of the Dead* is the conflict between the European American communities that dominate, divide and despoil the land and the predominantly Native, African American and Latino communities who have been dispossessed."[16] One character explains that the Europeans left their gods in Europe when they came to conquer the Americas. A deadly imitation of spirituality resulted, one that not only justified violent conquest (as well as destruction of the land and each other) but demanded it. This same character claims that, to their peril, Europeans do not know how to listen to the "souls of their dead": "Thus Europeans were haunted by the dead in their dream life and were driven mad by the incessant cries of unquiet ancestors' souls. No wonder they were such restless travellers; no wonder they wanted to go to Mars and Saturn" (604). But it is not only Euro-Americans who have lost belief in their past or their ancestors. Silko constructs indigenous characters who deny their heritage and emulate westerners with their idolatry of wealth and technology. Part of the complexity of *Almanac* arises from Silko's nonessentialist refusal to identify one group as evil and another as completely good. What Silko makes clear, however, is that those characters in the novel who distance themselves from their indigenous origins have also become the heartless, passionless machines of greed and destruction that *Almanac* accuses Euro-Americans of being.

Silko's disturbing and apocalyptic tale places medicine and science under the microscope of an unrelentingly critical gaze that foregrounds the distortions to which medicine is subject in a society obsessed with the gods of material gain and technological progress. The novel challenges readers to consider not only the individual's role but also the role of institutional ignorance, complicity, and neglect as factors contributing to oppression and disease. In *Almanac*, medicine is an enterprise as menacing to the poor as it is advantageous to the wealthy. *Almanac* does not, however, simply level a critique at medicine. Instead, it anatomizes the context in which medicine must do its work. The institution is both culpable *and* vulnerable. Unlike popular and science fiction novels that paint medicine's potential horrors in lurid colors, *Almanac* instead looks at the society medicine has helped create and within which it is trapped.

Almanac is difficult reading, however, precisely because it not only warns about and critiques technological progress but also insists on locating the roots of technological madness in the initial conquest of the Americas. Indeed, the history of technology itself has been, in its unchallenged state, a narrative of noble conquest—the conquest of "the enemy, whether it be human or the natural world—a narrative of progress, and of the betterment of humanity in general."[17] *Almanac*, however, undercuts the concept of technology as the noble conqueror. The malaise in *Almanac* represents (in the terms of psychoanalysis) a return of the repressed: the reality of violent conquest. Carefully constructed historical narratives have attempted to erase the brutality of this conquest. The violent roots of our national origins are, however, the palimpsest that continually disrupts notions of U.S. bedrock decency and democracy. The text suggests that the insanity and corruption represented in *Almanac* are simply the natural outcomes of two centuries of living with the psychic chasm that lies between the myth and rhetoric of religious/democratic foundations and the reality of violent conquest. The text implicates and embeds medicine in the conflict arising from the fruits of a progress that yields its spoils to a mere handful of the world's inhabitants and depends for its success on exploitation and oppression of the rest.[18]

Silko weaves several issues relevant to medicine throughout her elaborate textual web: the interrogation of medicine's profit motive; the commodification of the body (especially in the biomaterials business and in human organ transplantation, but in genetic technologies as well); the misuse of potentially healing technologies; the consequences of misplaced faith in technology; and the ways such faith turns on itself. Each of these issues stands in direct contrast to *Almanac*'s vision of an indigenous force (and its allies) that continually gathers strength for the earth's reclamation and healing.

One of the characteristics of the declining but dominant society created in *Almanac* is its ability to tolerate and maintain a patent disregard for human life and, while doing so, to make a sizable profit. *Almanac*'s narrator tells a story of sorcerers, or witches, who had once populated entire villages and who had pledged "to prey only on outsiders" and not on one another. They broke those pledges, however, and often "in the most bloodthirsty manner" as "brother killed brother [and] sister devoured sister." Indeed, "this destruction, this sorcery, this witchcraft, occurred among all human beings. The killing and devouring occurred behind bedroom doors, inflicted by parents and relatives, and the village of sorcerers continues generation after generation without interruption" (478). Chilling though this description may be, it hardly sounds like myth or ancient history. One only has to tune in to the nightly news to hear similar—and worse—stories. Genocide, ethnic cleansing, military occupation, domestic violence, and child abuse all continue to escalate while technological progress is virtually ineffectual in the face of these issues.

Silko's fable thus becomes a mirror for the sick world. And oddly enough, the sorcerers take on the characteristics of healers. The narrator notes that the sorcerers had gotten rich "making up and selling various odd sorts of 'tribal healing magics' and assorted elixirs, teas, balms, waters, crystals, and capsules to the city people, mostly whites [who] anxiously purchased indigenous cures for their dark nights of the soul on the continents where Christianity had repeatedly violated its own canons" (478). They sell these products, of course, at high prices, and aping what many medical practitioners would justly consider good biopsychosocial methods, "the sorcerers listened to the ailments and complaints of the city patients to gain knowledge of the patients' lives; the cures the sorcerers had then sold their 'patients' had cost hundreds, but consisted mostly of floor sweepings containing rodent dung and cotton lint" (479). Sorcery thus takes a leaf out of medicine's book, learning about the profit potential in disease and suffering. By linking sorcery's greed and charlatanism to medicine's profit-making aspects, as well as its laudable attempts to become more sensitive and aware of the contexts of patients' lives, the novel both implicates and warns contemporary medicine of the complicated and destructive marriage of greed and a technology that supposedly serves human life.

The concept that illness is big money especially fascinates Trigg, a minor character in *Almanac*. Trigg's wild enthusiasm for the profits he has made in the blood plasma and illegal organ harvest business and those profits that await him as the need (and possibility) for human organ transplants rise is not surprising. The demand for human organs in this country has grown exponentially with the dramatic advent of transplantation technology coupled with the discovery of immunosuppressive drugs such as cyclosporine in the 1970s and, later in the late 1980s (as cyclosporine's benefits were eclipsed by its side effects and failures), the development of FK 506.[19] Looking at a set of statistics on kidney transplantation, "the oldest and most often performed transplants," Renee Fox and Judith Swazey point out that in 1991 the number of patients waiting for cadaveric kidney transplantation increased monthly by 200. The authors of the study point out that 300 *additional* donors were needed per month to reverse the shortage crisis significantly, and 100 were needed simply to break even.[20] While the number of persons awaiting transplants has risen, the number of cadaveric donors, however, remains between sixteen and eighteen per million people (population).[21] In 1997, 4,000 people on transplantation waiting lists died waiting for an organ.[22]

Knowing what to do about these shortages is less simple than documenting them. In the United States, articles in scholarly journals run the gamut from recommendations to improve the current system for organ procurement to considerations of systems such as conscription (a type of organ "draft," not unlike our military draft);[23] compensation (where families of deceased persons are paid for the so-called donation); and a market system.[24] With organ markets, which most writers argue would be limited to cadaveric organs, potential donors or surviving family members would offer their organs for a market-determined price to procurement firms. Remuneration could take the form of lowered health insurance payments, burial insurance, or outright cash payments. Scholars have argued variously about the ethical problems inherent in all of these proposals.[25]

Silko's concerns about the commodification of bodies and the traffic in human organs are particularly significant in light of cases such as that of physician H. Barry Jacobs, founder and medical director of International Kidney Exchange, Inc. In 1983 Jacobs solicited 7,500 hospitals to enter a national and international marketing scheme through his company. Jacobs proposed "commissioning kidneys from persons living in the Third World or in disadvantaged circumstances in the United States for whatever price would induce them to sell their organs, and then negotiating their acquisition, for a fee, by Americans who could afford to purchase them."[26] More recently, in 1999 the *Chicago Sun-Times* ran a short article titled "eBay Halts Bidding for Kidney" when the bidding on an Internet auction site hit $5.7 million.[27] Recent debates about stem cell research crystallize current fear and desire at the same time around the issue of organ transplantation and prolongation of life through technology. It is hardly news that a lucrative market in illegal organ harvesting—a potential gold mine—lays at the ready or, recognizing this fact, that Silko makes use of it in her critique of modern medicine and contemporary society.

In *Almanac*, human bodies—and body parts—become just another high-yield market commodity. Hot sellers include not only human organs (hearts, livers, lungs, kidneys, and corneas) but fetal brain material, human skin for grafts, and of course, blood plasma. A brisk pornographic trade exists between the United States and South America, where videos of live torture, abortions, fetal dissections, human experiments, and surgical operations are made and sold. Sex-change surgeries and "ritual circumcisions of six year-old virgins" (103) are especially popular; one viewer is so thrilled, he is "afraid to feel how much he enjoyed the scalpel sinking through skin and flesh" (538).

Silko turns the commodification of the body back on the commodifier, however. For example, Eric, one of *Almanac*'s minor characters, commits suicide, distraught over his relationship with his lover, the photographer David. Upon hearing Eric's telephoned threat of suicide, David rushes to Eric, not to prevent the suicide, but to photograph its aftermath: "After discovering Eric's body, David didn't just snap a few pictures. He had moved reflectors around and got the light so Eric's blood appeared as bright and glossy as enamel paint. . . . Influential international critics agreed; at last David 'had found a subject to fit his style of clinical detachment and relentless exposure of what lies hidden in flesh'" (108). Clinical detachment and the medical gaze have run amok as they join the profit motive. The result is not simply that David can make Eric's blood look like enamel under his lights and with sophisticated technology, but that David's blood *itself* has turned as hard as the enamel he creates on Eric's body. *Almanac*'s milieu being what it is, these photographs make David a controversial but immediate sensation in the art world. If we were to change the subject from art to medical innovation (especially human organ transplantation), the issue becomes medicine's vulnerability, like David's, and the possibility of its turning to enamel, becoming hardened to the realities of human suffering in the excitement of technological innovation. David is a prime example of the witchery's fulfillment in *Ceremony*: to wrench the heart out of living human beings and leave them gutless, without feeling.

Similarly, the wealthy and aristocratic Argentinean Serlo is so obsessed with *sangre pura* that he dreams of creating a pure-blooded master race. "Serlo had *sangre pura*; 'blue blood' deserved 'blue blood.' In the end there could be nothing better" (542). Serlo, "the last and oldest boy virgin on the continent" (547), has dedicated himself to the cause of "upgrad[ing] mestizo and Indian bloodstock" (541). While Silko creates David as hardened in the face of death, she creates Serlo as a figure for loveless, sexless, mechanical reproduction. Disgusted by human sexual contact, "his sex organ touched only sterile, prewarmed stainless steel cylinders used for the artificial insemination of cattle." Serlo plans to use his extensive resources (both biological and financial) to develop an institute for research and experimentation in racial "upgrading."[28] Planning to obtain sperm donations from "European males of noble birth" (547), Serlo deeply fears that "brown people would inherit the earth like the cockroaches unless [he] and the others were successful at the institute" (561). Serlo predictably admires the Third Reich, since "there was little use in bringing a genetically superior man into a world crowded and polluted by the degenerate masses" (546), and he believes that the "common rabble" are fit only as organ donors (560). In fact, to Serlo, HIV is the ultimate "designer" virus, "specifically for targeted groups." With HIV, "the filthy would die" and the "clean would live." (Serlo no doubt would have applauded the deep ecologists' use of HIV-positive subjects as human bombs.) HIV, claims Serlo, is "the great biological bomb," the result of an international collaboration, first "detonated" in Africa, "where researchers hoped malnutrition would enhance the virus's power" (548).

Another character, Clinton, would have no trouble believing this. He is convinced that "illness, dope and hunger . . . [are] the white man's allies" because "only dope stopped young black men from burning white America to the ground" (426). In addition, Clinton makes the connection between the ecology movement and ethnic cleansing:

> Lately Clinton had seen ads purchased by so-called "deep ecologists." The ads blamed earth's pollution not on industrial wastes—hydrocarbons and radiation—but on overpopulation. It was no coincidence the Green Party originated in Germany. "Too many people" means "too many *brown-skinned* people." Clinton could read between the lines. "Deep ecologists" invariably ended their magazine ads with "Stop immigration!" and "Close the borders!" [415].

Thus Silko links illness, drugs, poverty, border patrol, and a potentially genocidal Green movement in one sweeping gesture. Clinton's assessment foregrounds the national unease with otherness and the sinister aspects of social control within a human community grown cold with the pursuit of wealth and technological advance.

In such a context, human beings are reduced to their marketable parts, the consequence of which is an easily rationalized commodification of the body that serves the social function of dealing with undesirables or, as Trigg writes in his journal, "human debris." Writing specifically about human organ transplantation, Patricia A. Marshall warns that

> the biomedical "gaze" . . . of organ transplantation technology fosters a view of the person as a disembodied entity. It is precisely this shift in orientation to the human body, and

to the person in the body, that heightens concerns for op-
ponents of a commoditization of human body parts. If the
body is viewed as marketable, the person is at risk of being
viewed as a commodity. This perspective exacerbates the
objectification of the human body that already exists in
biomedicine and sharpens the separation of the spiritual,
social, and mindful body from the physiological being.[29]

The commodified body, then, moves from an external (such as pros-
titution) to an internal (full of marketable parts) commodification
and, as such, becomes potential prey to medical technology and its
practitioners.

Zygmunt Bauman's notions of how modernist society deals with
the Other sheds light on the potential function of such commodification. Bauman characterizes modern society as one that is "anthropoemic," that is, one that "vomits" its enemies, or the Other, the not-
us. He contrasts this with Claude Lévi-Strauss's notion that older
societies were "anthropophagic," that is, they ate or ingested the
Other. Bauman argues that "our way of dealing with the Other (and,
thus, obliquely, of producing and re-producing our own identity) is to
segregate, separate, dump onto the rubbish tip, flush down into the
sewer of oblivion."[30] For Bauman, racist discourse and politics are
the "manifestations of mainly anthropoemic . . . strateg[lies] of modern order-maintenance."[31] How human organ transplantation might
function as such a strategy lies in the transformation of the organ-as-
gift into the organ-as-commodity. In their discussion of the trans-
action between donor and recipient, Fox and Swazey note, "At the
center of organ transplantation is a gift of surpassing significance. . . .
Paradoxically, it is an offering that so perfectly epitomizes one of the
ultimate Judeo-Christian values of our society—the injunction to
give ourselves to each other in ways that include our strangers as well
as our brothers and sisters—it transcends what is ordinarily asked or
expected of us."[32] The authors argue that as our society moves further from the gift mentality, we find it easier to think of transplantation in more value-neutral, biologized terms.[33]

Almanac's focus on human organ transplantation, however, constructs a closed loop containing both of what Bauman terms the anthropoemic and anthropophagic elements of order maintenance, for it is not *all* bodies that are rendered fodder for scientific and medical gain but, predictably, those that are deemed worthless (and Other) by the dominant society. In 1985 the Transplantation Society issued guidelines for the distribution and use of organs, pointing out what current news media report with some regularity:

> In a South American country . . . advertisements from desperate individuals have appeared in newspapers offering a kidney or even an eye (for corneal transplantation) for money. In this regard, many of us receive occasional pathetic appeals from people in disadvantaged countries offering to sell a kidney to get money, often for care of an ill relative. Besides being an eloquent comment on the social inequalities of our society in general, such appeals raise unsettling ethical questions of a more specific nature. . . . Furthermore, an active market of living unrelated kidney transplantation with payment to donors is occurring in at least one city in India; some of these donors make their way, with the potential recipient and "proof" of consanguinity, to the West. Thus recently, a major newspaper has described the buying of kidneys from impoverished donors for transplantation in private hospitals in Western countries. Some donations were coerced, some for meager fees; and allegedly there was no follow-up of the donors after surgery.[34]

With the escalation of ethnic cleansing throughout the world and the paranoid control of borders in the United States and elsewhere, the commerce in human bodies has a menacing pragmatism: getting rid of certain (radically unstable) categories of people, so-called undesirables (the anthropoemic function), and in so doing, creating the means to save those worth saving (with organ transplantation fulfilling the anthropophagic function).

Silko deepens her critique of contemporary society by suggesting that the connection between the commodification of body parts and medicine's profit motive is closely tied both to the idea of technological progress and to many forms of oppression. For example, *Almanac*'s Trigg, the owner of several blood plasma centers, buys many of his biomaterials in Mexico, where "recent unrest and civil strife had killed hundreds a week."[35] The unrest in Mexico—caused by the oppression of countless poor—is very much to Trigg's advantage because it will supply plenty of cadavers for organ harvesting, with only one problem: "Mexican hearts were lean and strong, but Trigg had found no market for dark cadaver skin" (404). Trigg figures that even if the war abated and cadavers became less available from Mexico, "hoboes or wetbacks could be 'harvested' at the plasma centers where a doctor had already examined the 'candidate' to be sure he was healthy" (663).[36]

Trigg, who has used a wheelchair since a spinal cord accident in college, provides perhaps the most egregious example of a predator who is legitimized by, supported by, and necessary to medicine. It is, however, Trigg's own precarious position as a potential social throwaway that adds to his virulence: he becomes what he fears. Early in his career Trigg writes, "breakthroughs in electrochemistry of the human brain. The rewiring of human nerves severed or badly crushed. Money buys anything. . . . Ike calls from West Germany. Says he's got a deal over there. They will buy all the blood and bioproducts we can deliver. Blood plasma centers are only the beginning" (386). Embedded in the euphoria over profit potential is the desperate hope that technology will find a way to heal his own "crushed nerves." In his college journals, for example, Trigg writes that he "feel[s] really stupid because the chair almost tips when I reach down for the notebook. . . . In the hospital I had dreams about walking and running. The chair is not me. The chair is not part of me" (384). Later he writes that his "dream goal" is "to walk down the aisle with my bride, not roll in this fucking chair" (385). Trigg's fascination with technology makes sense, but his detestation of his disability and the chair is testimony to the ways society has failed him. He can *only* trust technology in a social world where barriers are the norm for disabled people and where his social worth is just a slight remove from the "wetbacks and hoboes" he so hates. Trigg (and society) cannot see beyond the necessity for a cure (the need for technology at any cost) to look instead at the potential in creating a barrier-free world where people in wheelchairs (and blind or nonhearing people) would have equal access (and acceptance).

Trigg is, however, trapped in his social milieu and is also clearly an odious character. He supplies not only blood plasma but also other biomaterials, including human organs, to medical schools. With "the price quotes for fresh whole blood, human corneas and cadaver skin" buzzing in his head, Trigg has adroitly worked his connections with "human organ transplant research teams at the university hospital" (389). As the owner of a chain of plasma donor centers, Trigg has bought up the downtown area of Tucson "block by shabby block" in order to get it rezoned for his centers. It is not just that Trigg will make extraordinary profits from Blood Plasma International (and all that it involves), but as he brags to real estate mogul Leah Blue (who happens to be married to a professional broker of international assassinations), the "donor centers busted neighborhoods and drove property prices down without moving in blacks or Mexicans." This scheme allows Trigg to buy up the surrounding property at "forty cents on the dollar" (379).

Almanac suggests additional ways in which medicine's profits are used for the gain of the wealthy at the expense of the poor. Trigg recruits street people, hitchhikers, and drug addicts—all "disposable" human beings—to give blood at his center. Trigg hires Rambo Roy (Clinton's co-leader of the Army of the Homeless) to comb the parks and alleys for donors and pays him fifty cents for each person he brings in. Trigg has written of these so-called donors in his journal: "These alleged human beings, the filth and scum who pass through the plasma donor center, get paid good money for lying with a needle in their arms—an activity they pursue the rest of the day anyway. I could do the world a favor each week and connect a few of the stinking ones up in the back room and drain them dry. They will not be missed" (386). Trigg, in fact, does bleed several dry, using his centers to obtain organs and "other valuable human tissue" (387) that he sells illegally to West German consortia and to his "silent partners" in U.S. medical schools. Trigg confesses to Roy that he gets "excited" picking up hitchhikers as part of his harvesting methodology:

> He had thought of it as a roll of the dice or a hand of five-card draw. The winners and the discards. Discards were "locals" or those with too many kin. . . . Trigg had not minded the killing. . . . Trigg talked obsessively about the absence of struggle as the "plasma donors" were slowly bled to death pint by pint. A few who had attempted to get away had lost too much blood to put up much fight even against a man in a wheelchair. [444]

Trigg pays extra if the victim puts up no struggle and agrees to the procedure, giving him "a blow job while his blood fill[s] pint bags." The victim relaxes in the chair, "unaware he was being murdered." For Trigg, the "donors" are nothing but "human refuse," of whom "only a few had organs of sufficient quality for transplant use" (444).

Trigg understands that it is not, after all, therapeutic drugs any more, but biomaterials ("the industry's 'preferred' term for fetal-brain material, human kidneys, hearts and lungs, corneas for eye transplants, and human skin for burn victims") that will "be the bonanza of the twenty-first century" (398). Progressive technologies such as a recently available saline gel developed by the Japanese to keep human organs "fresh-frozen and viable for transplants for months, not hours," add to the bliss of possibility for Trigg (404). In his character, Silko brings together her critique of medicine's profit motive, its uncritical reliance on the power of technology, and its reproduction of oppressive systems, behaviors, and attitudes. Through commodification of the body (and its internal parts), medicine becomes a principal agent in segregating and ingesting "human debris" as a way of maintaining a pernicious form of social order.

For those who have wealth, there is even more money to be made from illness and suffering. Trigg's vision of creating his own medical conglomerate in southern Arizona—a hospital, an ambulance service, a mortuary, and housing developments for the disabled (soft money might be available from the government) as well as "fat farms" and the always profitable alcohol and drug treatment centers—comes close to suggesting corporate medicine. For Trigg, "the health care industry is a sleeping giant" that he proposes to awaken to fabulous financial gain: "There were millions and millions to be made" (382). After afternoons of sex, Trigg and Leah dream of ways to make ever more profits. Trigg argues constantly that the big money will be found not in real estate but in the medical and biomaterials industries. In fact, Trigg finally convinces Leah to join him in his medical schemes:

> Leah was on track about a medical hospital. They could build the facility near the detox-rehab hospital. They would need a regular hospital from time to time for their detox patients. Leah had got the idea for a kidney dialysis machine that would serve the sector of town houses and condominiums that would presumably be bought by kidney patients and their families or by health insurers to house their Arizona dialysis patients. [387]

Like a blight, Trigg's schemes grow as he develops plans for his medical complex (and a sex or "pleasure" mall for clients well enough to enjoy it). Even though the State of Arizona is collapsing (and therefore cheaply to be bought), terminally ill patients, in their misery, would not notice or mind the thousands of homeless people sleeping in Tucson's arroyos and streets. Nor would they care about being in such close proximity to Mexico's civil wars and the flood of immigrants pouring into Arizona. Setting his sights not only on terminally ill patients, though, Trigg plans for Tucson to become an international center for research, organ transplants, and cosmetic surgery (the beauty of which is that "when the fat came off or was sucked out, yards and yards of sagging wattles and crepey skin remained to be snipped off or tucked" [663]).

Not only obsessed with the financial returns from his bio-enterprises but also driven by the certainty that medical technology would progress far enough in his lifetime to heal his spinal cord injury and allow him to walk again, Trigg has, like many characters in the novel, an unwavering faith in technology as *the* redemptive force in contemporary society.[37] Yet neither his wealth nor his belief in the power of technology can ultimately save Trigg. When Leah Blue hears that Trigg has been murdered, her first thought is that the transplant doctors had finally gotten him. "Trigg used to say not even the lowest street addicts were as greedy as surgeons. His 'silent partners' at the medical school had made millions with their heart and lung transplant racket, but routinely they had accused Trigg of skimming profits" (751). Trigg is, in fact, murdered by his procurer, Rambo Roy, who incidentally swears that one of the first things the Army of the Homeless will do after the revolution is to accuse the biomaterials business of mass murder. The point here is not simply that Trigg and the doctors are corrupt (although they are), but that medicine's faith in technology is dangerously misplaced. Without the moral vision to employ the technology in solidarity with and on behalf of the oppressed of the world, those people most vulnerable in our world will continue to be exploited—and the exploiters will continue to self-destruct.

This unfailing trust in technology becomes a key element in the ongoing self-destruction of Euro-Americans and others who have left their heritage behind. For example, Menardo is a Mexican Indian who has worked hard to distance himself from his people and his past. He is the multimillionaire owner of Universal Insurance. Universal (with its name that begs the question, "for whom?") claims to protect the interests of Mexico's elite against theft, vandalism, and natural disasters as well as an ever-present threat of revolution and insurrection. But Menardo the insurer begins to realize there is no insurance that can protect his life, and he becomes completely fixed on the (perceived) powers of a bullet-proof vest given to him by his client, Max Blue (husband of Leah). Violent nightmares and the dread of death haunt Menardo. Wearing the vest, however (even while sleeping), he feels a sense of security, albeit a fragile one. Enthralled—obsessed—with the vest's presumed powers and planning to impress his friends, he eventually orders his indigenous chauffeur, Tacho (El Feo's brother), to fire a gun at him while he wears the vest. "Menardo wanted perfect timing—he wanted Tacho to wait until the cars had pulled up, then he would greet his fellow shooting-club members, then Tacho must shoot. Snap! Snap! Snap! One two three! Before the others could even open their mouths! What an exhibition they would see! Here was a man to be reckoned with—a man invincible with the magic of high technology" (503). What follows is later billed as a "freak accident." When Tacho reluctantly shoots the pathetic Menardo, the vest fails to protect him: "Microscopic imperfections in the fabric's quilting; a bare millimeter's difference and the bullet would safely have been stopped" (509). Menardo's arrogance and complete trust in technology's powers of protection become an example of Silko's witchery turning on itself.

The circumstances of Menardo's death anticipate the story of the "Ghost Shirts," told much later in the novel by activist-poet Wilson Weasel Tail at the International Holistic Healers Convention. Weasel Tail tells how the Europeans became disillusioned when they discovered that these shirts had not really protected their people from death, as promised by the Native Americans. Weasel Tail explains that "the anthropologists, who feverishly sought magic objects to postpone their own deaths had misunderstood the power of the ghost shirts. Bullets of lead belong to the everyday world; ghost shirts belong to the realm of spirits and dreams. The ghost shirts gave the dancers spiritual protection while the white men dreamed of shirts that repelled bullets because they feared death" (722). Menardo has a terror of death, like the white anthropologists, as well as a fear of being identified as indigenous, and he trusts only in the white man's bullet-proof vest while he fails to understand (and actively derides) the kind of protection that could help him, that which would come from a culturally rooted spiritual source. The trust in technology and the denial of his ancestors and spiritual roots are symptomatic of what Menardo's grandfather had termed (when Menardo was young and still in touch with his family) the temporary reign of "Death-Eye Dog" currently in force in the Americas. Death and destruction characterize the epoch in which the "orphan" Europeans (as well as those orphaned from their Indian heritage) are compelled to kill one another and destroy the earth as well (258). Menardo's trust in the vest undoes him, as does absolute trust in any technology, the novel suggests.

For example, in a frightening scene, an Alaskan Yupik woman uses the "old ways" to outwit modern aerodynamics:

> White people could fly circling objects in the sky that sent messages and images of nightmares and dreams, but the old woman knew how to turn the destruction back on its senders. . . . The old woman had gathered great surges of energy out of the atmosphere, by summoning spirit beings through recitations of the stories that were also indictments of the greedy destroyers of the land. With the stories the old woman was able to assemble powerful forces flowing from the spirits of ancestors. [156]

These powerful forces allow the Yupik woman to work a plane-crashing spell by rubbing a special weasel pelt on a TV screen that displays the weather channel as she intones a tragic story from the community's collective past. The screen fills with interference, and then a picture: "The pilot descends, then climbs and descends again, searching for a hole, searching for a break in the fog he entered only a minute earlier. The needle of the compass whirls and shivers in magnetic fields of false and true north. The altimeter is frozen at 2,000 and nothing can dislodge it. The copilot works frantically. . . . Then the screen goes white" (157). It is no accident that the owner of the crashed plane is the "largest single insurer of petroleum exploration companies in Alaska" (159). Those whom technology has oppressed learn to appropriate the technology, creating a micrograph of what will happen on a global level if things do not change. For a society committed to oppressive practice, there can be no insurance, the novel warns. The people themselves will rise up against the most sophisticated weapons and tools. In its completely improbable manner, the source of change will arrive through the dispossessed.

Nothing in *Almanac* brings good news to medicine. The novel forces readers to grapple with the purposes and uses of scientific and medical progress as it exists in a cruel and unjust world.[38] Silko refuses to absolve institutions from complicity in oppression and insists that they are accountable to the community and society in which they exist. As such, institutions are also at risk for or vulnerable to manipulation purely for profit, as Trigg's use of medicine well illustrates. Although Silko provides readers with few answers, the characters who are not hopelessly corrupt are those who are willing to listen to improbable voices—like those of the prophetic macaws that lead Tacho and El Feo, along with a growing Native American group traveling northward; the exhortations of Wilson Weasel Tail or the Barefoot Hopi ("he talked about the dead as if their spirits still hovered among the living" [625]); or the inner voice that prompts Sterling, an exiled Laguna, to return to his native land and rejoin his community. In *Almanac*, the struggle seems to be to wrest one's light from the deep shadows of a modern technological hell and find the courage to act in accordance with that light. As one reviewer notes, the larger context of *Almanac* is "that the apocalypse of the rapacious is at hand and that coalitions are formed by those who act."[39]

What of the "silent partners" of Trigg's schemes, the medical schools? George Annas writes about self-deception in questing for what he calls the Holy Grail in medical experimentation. The issue could hold for such a complex matter as human organ transplantation, which is doubly complicated by its market-driven value and its human life-giving value. "Changing our ways in our postmodern world will not be easy. Our quest for the Holy Grail of medicine (immortality?), as honorable as it is in theory, can become destructive in practice."[40] The banality of evil that speaks through the simple words, "I'm just doing my job," and refuses to look at the broader issues in that doing is relevant to the deadening world *Almanac* constructs. Silko's novel behooves us to ask where human rights and civil rights issues are addressed in medical school curricula. When bioethics so frequently deals with individual patient decisions, it seems urgent to broaden the scope to include such foci, for example. *Almanac* specifically challenges medicine to consider its choices and actions in a social milieu that is potentially and profoundly destructive, not only to the poor and vulnerable, but to medicine itself. The question is whether medicine will risk listening to the improbable voices it can hear if it stops to listen, and how it will institutionally gather forces for its own healing, as well as for the difficult work of healing its patients. The *how* of that move forward is always complicated and is not the responsibility of institutionalized medicine and health care workers alone. As medicine sees itself as an accountable member of the human community—the global community—perhaps new ways of doing and seeing will render it less vulnerable to the greed and corruption of characters like Trigg.

Almanac of the Dead, complicating the notion of progress, bids readers to look carefully at connections, complicated and messy, among technological progress (such as the increased capacity for organ transplantation); our assumptions about borders (who belongs? why? who, after all, is an American and what difference does it make?); our assumptions about worthiness and unworthiness; and how those assumptions are linked to pernicious and tenacious foundations of racism, ethnocentrism, homophobia, classism, and sexism. Medicine is inextricably bound to the ongoing enterprise of oppression and domination. It is that link, the novel insists, that allows medicine to be corrupted—infected—by the likes of Trigg, who will, for a profit, serve the double purposes of ridding the country of undesirables and providing their organs for those deemed worthy, or Menardo, who believes technology will provide the antidote to death. As long as medicine functions ignorantly within the corrupting and corrupted social systems of the Americas, it too, Silko warns, will remain both diseased and infectious.

A Dream of *Communitas*

Octavia Butler's *Parable of the Sower* and *Parable of the Talents* and Roads to the Possible

8

> In the bruising fist of challenge
> the future does not tarry.
> —Audre Lorde, "Prism"

> And it is a kind of hunger
> that brings us to love.
> —Linda Hogan, "Hunger"

The scenarios Silko creates in *Almanac of the Dead* seem almost civilized next to the worlds of Octavia Butler's *Parable of the Sower* and *Parable of the Talents*, novels set primarily in the not-so-distant years of 2015–35.[1] Using elements of various genres, including slave and freedom narratives, diaries, realist fiction, survivalist stories, and religious prose and poetry, Butler creates a world that bears many similarities to our own, only worse. It is a world in which systems of public service are rendered completely ineffective, humans prey on one another, and lawlessness seems to be the only rule—except for the wealthiest who can afford to buffer themselves from the rest of society. In the world of *Sower* and *Talents*, even the middle class cannot survive behind walled communities and sophisticated technologies (that are mostly defunct because of power shortages or prohibitive costs).

While Butler's novels are usually considered science fiction, *Parable of the Sower* and *Parable of the Talents* also contain strong elements of critical dystopian fiction and realism. The voice in these novels Hoda Zaki characterizes as "prophetic [and] dystopian."[2] While Stephen Potts describes *Parable of the Sower* as a novel that is "fundamentally about social power," the same can be said of *Parable of the Talents*.[3] Although *Sower* and *Talents* are not science fiction in the same way that Butler's Patternist or Xenogenisis series are (there are no three-gendered rescuers from other universes, no disease-mutated people with superhuman abilities), there are monsters. These are the all-too-human monsters created by greed, neglect, and stupidity. Some are drug-induced monsters. Many of the monsters—in fact, the majority in *Talents*—are in power and are clean-cut, religious, "moral leaders." These novels draw on elements of science fiction, creating a world of both horror and beauty, demanding that readers grapple with alternatives to the horror. Mehaffy and Keating ask, "In its unorthodox *formal* aesthetics, how much political power and efficacy might Butler's science fiction, or any radical author's fiction, promise as a revisionary social project?"[4] Indeed, Butler tells Mehaffy and Keating that both novels represent cautions about the "dangers of a fundamentalist religion-driven national politics, as exemplified in Pat Robertson's 1992 run for the U.S. presidency, and about the climate changes, emblematized by global warming, occurring in the two fictional landscapes and in contemporary real time." But she also states that she wanted to go further than warning, and thus through the spiritual vision and leadership of her main character, Lauren, Butler explores how human attitudes might be changed in terms of how we treat one another and Earth.[5]

Tom Moylan argues that Butler's *Parable of the Sower* can be read as a critical dystopia because it "continue[s] in the political and poetic spirit of the critical utopias even as [it] revive[s] the dystopian strategy to map, warn, and hope."[6] Partly answering Mehaffy and Keating's earlier question, he says, "Dystopian narrative is largely the product of the terrors of the twentieth century," and he asserts that it has the "ability to register the impact of an unseen and unexamined social system on the everyday lives of everyday people."[7] Moylan goes further, however, and looks at critical dystopia as a "textual mutation that self-reflexively takes on the present system and offers not only astute critiques of the order of things but also explorations of the oppositional spaces and possibilities from which the next round of political activism can derive imaginative sustenance and inspiration."[8] Indeed, both *Sower* and *Talents* at once critique and seek transformational possibilities in a textual world where Butler has left few such possibilities available. She calls on readers to stretch the limits of their own imaginative thinking and to push beyond the boundaries of what the texts present and the repressive politics in which we live today and, like Lauren, imagine the unimaginable.

The novels are, in part, about Lauren Olamina's evolution into a remarkable spiritual leader, but they are also about a rite of passage for an entire community. As the social structures disintegrate, something new emerges, fragile but innovative and durable. The novels dismantle the cultural myth of individualism, where one is responsible for both one's success and one's misfortune, and place both in a broader social context. The oppression, indeed the horrors Lauren and her multiracial, multiethnic community experience have historical roots that date back to slavery, classical religious mind-body dualism, colonialism (past and present), Puritanism, and more.[9] Butler, novelizing the concerns of scholars such as Dorothy Roberts, Susan Sherwin, and Howard Waitzkin, never lets readers forget that the personal troubles of individuals are rooted in much larger social and political realities. In addition, Butler's novels sketch broad outlines of a rite of passage into something new, an envisioning of alternative ways of thinking and being that are particularly illuminating and provocative when one considers medicine in the twenty-first century.

Victor Turner discusses rites of passage as points of transition, citing Van Gennep's three phases of passage: "separation, margin (or *limen*, signifying 'threshold' in Latin), and aggregation."[10] It is the marginal, or liminal, phase with which I am most interested. Turner argues that this is a period in which "the characteristics of the ritual subject (the 'passenger') are ambiguous; he passes through a cultural realm that has few or none of the attributes of the past or coming state."[11] This space constitutes the ground of radical instability, a place of unknowing, where what Turner calls *communitas* may emerge. Further, Turner opposes *communitas* to structural ties: "These are the ties organized in terms either of caste, class, or rank hierarchies."[12] *Communitas* includes a sacred component: "Something of the sacredness of that transient humility and modelessness goes over, and tempers the pride of the incumbent of a higher position or office," which in turn makes the space wherein "an essential and generic human bond" is recognized.[13] While Turner focuses on traditional preindustrial societies, he argues that it is clear that *communitas* may "be found at all stages and levels of culture and society."[14] Turner describes *communitas* as "a relationship between concrete, historical, idiosyncratic individuals . . . [who] are not segmentalized into roles and statuses, but confront one another rather in the manner of Martin Buber's 'I and Thou.' "[15]

For individuals, this happens as a result of inhabiting the liminal state, perhaps even a state of being unmoored from the familiar. I think of Myra Jehlen's argument that it was not until Huck Finn cross-dressed as a girl and was radically destabilized in terms of his gender—"plung[ed] . . . into the deepest possible limbo of identity"— that he was (shortly thereafter) able, momentarily, to associate himself fully with Jim as a fellow human being (rather than seeing him as an enslaved black man—an Other).[16] As individuals experience liminality or states of destabilization and lose their moorings, they may (and do, according to Turner's model) emerge with a new sense of being connected with others. Velma Henry, Ciel Turner, Avey Johnson, Tayo, Precious Jones, Cleófilas, and many of the other characters in the novels I have read for this study move through painful individualistic spaces into a time of instability, of what Turner would call "modelessness," and emerge with a new and empowering connection to community.

It seems to me, however, that it is possible to think beyond rites of individual passage and envision, much as I have with *Almanac of the Dead*, medicine itself as an entity with an undeveloped or unacknowledged potential for *communitas*, moving through a sort of institutional rite of passage, presently existing in its own liminal space where what was sure in the past is no longer, and what will be in the future is radically in question. What medicine's fulfillment of the World Health Organization's ample vision of health will be remains to be seen. More now than when, in 1986, the organization first enlarged the scope of health to include "the state of complete physical, mental and social well-being and not merely the absence of disease or infirmity,"[17] the challenges facing health care practitioners are, quite simply, overwhelming (not to mention the other side of the problematic: the possibility of medical authority—emphasis on authority— having far too great a sphere of influence in human existence). Additionally, not only does the scope of health change under this definition, but "the roles and responsibilities of health professionals and their relationship to the larger society"[18] also become radically expanded. Problematics notwithstanding, change is inevitable. How it happens and what kind of change it will be is not so inevitable.

Both *Parable of the Sower* and *Parable of the Talents* are novels about a dying society and change within it. They are also about a rite of passage that is arguably not all that far removed from our own society's transition into and through the twenty-first century. As Stephen Potts notes about *Sower*, the novel is "a close extrapolation from current trends: the increasing class gap, the fear of crime, the chaos of the cities spreading to the suburbs, the centrifugal forces tearing our society apart."[19] Indeed, writes Lauren Olamina in her "Earthseed: The Books of the Living," *God is change*, words that thread themselves throughout Butler's narratives. Not only is Lauren's god change, but

> God is Infinite,
>> Irresistible,
>> Inexorable,
>> Indifferent.
>> God is Trickster,
>>> Teacher,
>>> Chaos,
>>> Clay—

> God is Change.
> Beware:
> God exists to shape
> And to be shaped. [*Talents,* 49]

As Lauren Olamina's spiritual notations demonstrate, her theology is one of dynamic change. She moves radically from her father's Baptist preachings to construct a theology where humans are principally agents of change in a dynamic universe that exists to be shaped. Lauren's middle name is, in fact, Oya, the name of a Nigerian Orisha of the Yoruba people. "A dynamic, dangerous entity," writes Lauren's bitter daughter, wondering what her grandfather had seen in Lauren that he would have given her such a middle name, adding that Oya was also goddess of "the wind, fire, and death, more bringers of great change" (*Talents,* 50). The community that exists in *Sower* is clearly dying, and the frightening efforts to resuscitate it in *Talents* by way of a repressive and corrupt religious fundamentalism that includes slavery as one of its mechanisms of social control make it hard to imagine a space within which *communitas* might exist, but it is within the absolute upheaval—the liminality that makes change possible—that Earthseed is born.

Parable of the Sower begins in the year 2024. Fifteen-year old Lauren Olamina lives with her siblings, African American father, and Latina stepmother. Lauren, along with being precocious and extremely bright, is afflicted with hyperempathy syndrome. Lauren's birth mother had been addicted to Paracetco, a drug that caused Lauren's condition. Paracetco had been the

> popular "smart drug" of [Lauren's mother's] time. It was a
> new prescription medicine . . . and it was doing wonders
> for people who had Alzheimer's disease. It stopped the de-
> terioration of their intellectual function and enabled them
> to make excellent use of whatever memory and thinking
> ability they had left. It also boosted the performance of

> ordinary, healthy young people. They read faster, retained
> more, made more rapid, accurate connections, calcula-
> tions, and conclusions. As a result, Paracetco became as
> popular as coffee among students, and, if they meant to
> compete in any of the highly paid professions, it was as
> necessary as a knowledge of computers. [*Talents*, 18]

The drug is addictive; thousands of people die trying to break the habit, and it may have been the cause of the death of Lauren's mother when Lauren is born. The drug clearly leaves its mark on her (and millions of others like Lauren), manifested in hyperempathy syndrome. Popularly, Lauren is known as a "sharer"; she feels the agony of others when she sees them in pain or hears their cries (she also shares sexual pleasure, but as a preacher's daughter in an enclosed community, there is little of that to be had). Physicians call it "organic delusional syndrome," to which the young Lauren says, "Big shit. It hurts, that's all I know" (*Talents*, 10–11).[20]

Living in a world that can only be characterized as savagely at war with itself, Lauren is bombarded with sensations of violent pain everywhere she goes. When she shoots a wounded dog as a mercy killing, she feels "the impact of the bullet as a hard, solid blow—something beyond pain. Then I felt the dog die. . . . It went out like a match in a sudden vanishing of pain" (*Sower*, 39). Later in the novel, Lauren has to stab an attacker and feels every moment of it: "The six inch blade went in up to the hilt. Then, in empathic agony, I jerked it out again. I can't describe the pain" (*Sower*, 210). Lauren evokes the profundity of pain by denying the ability of language to conjure it. When Lauren's brother Keith is horribly tortured and killed ("someone had cut and burned away most of my brother's skin" [*Sower*, 100]), she imagines that if hyperempathy syndrome were more common, "people couldn't do such things. They could kill if they had to, and bear the pain of it or be destroyed by it. But if everyone could feel everyone else's pain, who would torture? Who would cause anyone unnecessary pain? . . . A biological conscience is better than no conscience at all," she muses (*Sower*, 102).

Her family's home in the mostly African American and Latino community of Robledo, twenty miles from Los Angeles, is located, like virtually all communities in *Sower* that house the middle class, behind a wall, "a massive, looming presence" Lauren sees as "a crouching animal, perhaps about to spring, more threatening than protective" (*Sower*, 5). Indeed, Robledo's inhabitants commonly encounter human corpses immediately beyond its walls. At times people will toss "gifts of envy" over the wall: "a maggoty, dead animal, a bag of shit, even an occasional severed human limb or a dead child" (*Sower*, 43). Lauren and her family hear gunfire day and night, "single shots and odd bursts of automatic weapons fire" and even heavy artillery blasts. Home is "an island surrounded by sharks" (*Sower*, 44). Refugees of those communities where walls have been destroyed and invaded clog highways and expressways. Going outside is to venture into the place "where things are so dangerous and crazy" (*Sower*, 6) and must be attempted only in well-armed and organized groups. Lauren sees a woman, "young, naked, and filthy" with a "slack expression" that suggests "she was dazed or drunk or something." But perhaps "she had been raped so much that she was crazy." The nearby canyon is littered with half-eaten corpses. The poorer communities are walled with "unmortared rocks, chunks of concrete, and trash," but the worst "were the pitiful, unwalled residential areas" that had mostly been "burned, vandalized, infested with drunks or druggies or squatted-in by homeless families with their filthy, gaunt, half-naked children" (*Sower*, 8). Fires are epidemic, thanks to the newest street drug, "pyro," that makes people crave fire and become both sexually aroused and satisfied by watching both the fire and its aftermath.

Stopping to offer aid to people in this society becomes an act of stupidity, since to do so is to risk being attacked by the hundreds of scavengers and drug-crazed people who live in the streets. "On the street, people are expected to fear and hate everyone but their own kind" (*Sower*, 31). Lauren understands the connection between poverty and the rampant spread of disease: The street poor "cut off each other's ears, arms, legs. . . . carry untreated disease and festering wounds. They have no money to spend on water to wash with, so even the unwounded have sores. They don't get enough to eat so they're malnourished—or they eat bad food and poison themselves" (*Sower*, 9). All communities suffer this breakdown of civilization, not just the poor. The rich are more buffered, but the trajectory is toward ruin for all, just as Lauren's relatively safe and barricaded community learns.

The technology so idolized by characters such as Trigg and Menardo in *Almanac of the Dead* is highly developed but useless, since no one can afford to use it. Electricity is a rarity, and city lights are a thing of the past. "All we have left now are three small, ancient, murky little TV sets scattered around the neighborhood, a couple of computers used for work, and radios" (*Sower*, 17). Sewage systems will not tolerate toilet paper, and all but expensive purified water is undrinkable. Weather conditions are chaotic. "Tornadoes are smashing hell out of Alabama, Kentucky, Tennessee, and two or three other states. Three hundred people dead so far. And there's a blizzard freezing the northern midwest, killing even more people. In New York and New Jersey, a measles epidemic is killing people" because no one can afford immunizations (*Sower*, 47). Later, cholera epidemics, hepatitis, and dengue—tropical diseases brought by the shifting weather—plague an ill-prepared nation.

Unemployment is rampant, and the president plans to change laws that keep the "restrictive" minimum wage in place, mandating worker protection laws "for those employers willing to take on homeless employees and provide them with training and adequate room and board." Lauren wonders about the notion of adequacy: "A house or apartment? A room? A bed in a shared room? A barracks bed? Space on a floor? Space on the ground? And what about people with big families? Won't they be seen as bad investments? Won't it make much more sense for companies to hire single people, childless couples, or, at most, people with only one or two kids?" (*Sower*, 24). When KSF, a German, Japanese, and Canadian company, takes over a dying small coastal town, Lauren believes that "something old and nasty is reviving" (*Sower*, 105). KSF privatizes the entire town, obtaining in the process "an eager, educated work force" with limited options (*Sower*, 106). For Lauren and her father, KSF spells slavery: "Get people into debt, hang on to them, and work them harder" (*Sower*, 107). In an interesting narrative move, Butler uses Lauren to comment on the way science fiction frequently has functioned prophetically: "Cities controlled by companies are old hat in science fiction. My grandmother left a whole bookcase of old science fiction novels. The company-city subgenre always seemed to star a hero who outsmarted, overthrew, or escaped 'the company.' I've never seen one where the hero fought like hell to get taken in and underpaid by the company. In real life, that's the way it will be. That's the way it is" (*Sower*, 110). *Parable of the Sower* may belong to the genre of science fiction, but using Lauren to critique the genre, Butler contests "shelving" her work and insists that her character's observations are based in urgent social and political realities, are a form of prophetic utterance.

Indeed, five years later, in *Parable of the Talents*, indenturing the poor is fashionable (and sounds a bit like our current welfare reform policies): "Indenturing indigents is supposed to keep them employed, teach them a trade, feed them, house them, and keep them out of trouble. In fact, it's just one more way of getting people to work for nothing or almost nothing" (*Talents*, 42–43). Not only economic slavery, but sexual slavery is viable as well. Men with incomes pick up homeless women and create polygamous families, limited only by how many women a man can afford to feed. Or a man will have one wife and several servant girls who function as a harem, and he might throw them out if they become pregnant.

Lauren has been both a visionary and a survivalist from a young age, and she gets into trouble for it. She makes connections between the bubonic plague in Europe and the contemporary situation. As a teenager, Lauren believes that if the survivors of such horrors as the bubonic plague in medieval Europe knew that change was real and could demand different working conditions, so too could their community in Robledo embrace change and become survivors (or wait to die). Lauren studies books on survival in the wilderness, guns and shooting, medical emergencies, native and naturalized plants and their uses, and basic living skills (such as log cabin construction, raising livestock, plant cultivation, and soap making). She puts together an emergency "grab and run pack" filled with food, clothing, money, matches, a blanket, seeds, and water (*Sower*, 51). Her father and his congregation (he is a minister as well as a college professor) are not pleased with what they consider her alarmist ideas. They think she is plotting to run away with her friend, and Lauren's father makes her swear not to talk about her prognostications and survival plans with anyone else because she is frightening the community, especially the other parents. She refuses to honor his demand until he agrees to suggest that community and congregation members begin preparing "earthquake packs" in case of natural disasters. In the meantime, Lauren and her father quietly bury provisions in plastic containers in the backyard.

One day Lauren's father does not return from his office at the college. Lauren joins the search party and sees "more squalor, more human remains, more feral dogs" than ever and notes the progression of social decay and peril. She never finds her father, but she does find an arm, a "black man's arm, just the color of my father's . . . slashed and cut all over" (*Sower*, 116). The searchers also see "the rotting corpses of five people . . . the cold remains of a fire with a human femur and two human skulls lying among the ashes" (*Sower*, 118) as well as a living child being eaten by dogs. Like the witchery in Silko's *Ceremony*, it is a dismembering evil, both literally and spiritually, that permeates Lauren's social world— indeed society as a whole. This evil seeks to cut individuals away from community and is characterized by the worse-than-animal behavior of humans against one another. Dismemberment also becomes dys-memory, the sense of being utterly cut off from any memory of something beyond the self's immediate hungers, but Lauren's vision for a better world, for something different from what she and her family experienced in Robledo and that she experiences beyond, includes a community of memory.

Lauren's father had been a leader in the community, and his death is felt as a tremendous loss. At his memorial service, Lauren preaches powerfully, articulating her nascent vision of a better world:

> "Those nightmares of mine are our future if we fail one an-
> other," I said, winding up. "Starvation, agony at the hands
> of people who aren't human any more. Dismemberment.
> Death. We have God and we have each other. We have our
> island community, fragile, and yet a fortress. Sometimes it
> seems too small and too weak to survive. And like the
> widow in Christ's parable, its enemies fear neither God nor
> man. But also like the widow, it persists. *We persist.*"
> [*Sower*, 120; emphasis in original]

Lauren figures hope as a persistent force that can be destroyed but resurrected. She writes in "The Books of the Living,"

> In order to rise
> From its own ashes
> A phoenix
> First
> Must
> Burn. [*Sower*, 137]

In this case, fire is the purification that begins the process of forward movement and change. When fire destroys Robledo and most of its residents, Lauren escapes with her "grab and run" pack and meets Zarah, one of Richard Moss's formerly homeless and starving co-wives. Moss had died in the violence during the fire, and Lauren ruefully notes that Zarah has gone from "nothing to nothing" in six years (*Sower*, 151). They run into another former neighbor, Harry, and the three decide to band together; Lauren dresses as a man for further protection. The freeway is filled with pedestrians, bicyclers, and people pushing carts. For safety, almost no one eats while walking because of the many predators (human and animal). Dogs are wild and eat babies and corpses. Everyone is visibly armed, and most people usually carry hidden weapons as well.

The radical space of *communitas* is that place of unknowing and uncertainty, that environment in which Lauren and her fellow travelers find themselves. Lauren writes,

> Earthseed
> Cast on new ground
> Must first perceive
> That it knows nothing. [*Sower*, 160]

Those who want to survive must

> Embrace diversity.
> Unite—
> Or be divided,
> robbed,
> ruled,
> killed
> By those who see you as prey.
> Embrace diversity
> Or be destroyed. [*Sower*, 176]

On an unlikely pilgrimage to an unknown destination, Lauren, Zarah, and Harry constitute a nightmare version of *The Canterbury Tales*, telling stories about their lives as they begin to trust one another. They learn radical trust as a means of survival. However, paradox is the order of the day. They also must learn a new way of being with other people—radical distrust as a method of survival. When they stop at commercial water stations, for example, two of them must watch with weapons in full view while the other fills the water jug. Persons who do not buy from the exorbitantly expensive water stations purchase their water from peddlers and are sometimes killed by the organisms or the "fuel, pesticide, herbicide, whatever else has been in the bottles that peddlers [who sometimes poison even themselves] use" (*Sower*, 180).

Lauren develops—discovers—Earthseed and the idea of a new community whose ultimate destiny lies in settling new frontiers in the stars, as she journeys through this dangerous and tenuous space with her unlikely companions and is joined by a few others. "Earthseed is about preparing to fulfill the Destiny. It's about learning to live in partnership with one another in small communities, and at the same time, working out a sustainable partnership with our environment. It's about treating education and adaptability as the absolute essentials that they are" (*Talents*, 322). Among those who join the group are Allison and Jill, two young women who had been prostitutes (pimped by their father), and a fifty-seven-year-old widowed family practice physician, Taylor Franklin Bankole.

Bankole lost his wife to a gang of thugs who beat her to get drugs (she had heart medication, and they also knew Bankole was a physician). She was so badly beaten he could not save her, especially since the robbers had taken the medicines, and the ambulance took more than an hour to arrive at the house. Despite their age differences (Lauren is eighteen), they form a bond through their mutual losses and the fact that both are descended from men who took and passed on African names to them. When Lauren tells Bankole about her hyperempathy syndrome, he offers her pain medications—not for herself, but for those who are experiencing the pain. (His advice is not unlike what a queasy intern might hear when confronted with a patient whose intense suffering threatens to eclipse the student's ability to work on that patient: "I'll teach you how and when to use [the drugs] on me or whoever needs them," says Bankole, adding, "If you can just hold on and be yourself long enough to use them, you can do whatever else may be necessary" (*Sower*, 250). To Bankole's comment about her syndrome, Lauren responds, "It might not be so bad a thing if most people had to endure all the pain they caused. Not doctors or other medical people, of course, but most people." Lauren adds that "self-defense shouldn't have to be an agony or a killing or both" (*Sower*, 249).

Emery Tanaka Solis, "the most racially mixed [person] that [Lauren] had ever met" (*Sower*, 258), who had a Japanese father, black mother, and Mexican husband, also joins the group. All of Emery's family has died except her nine-year-old daughter, Tori Solis. Emery's story illustrates the kind of slavery Lauren fears. A large agribusiness conglomerate bought the farm on which Emery and her family had worked in exchange for food, shelter and hand-me-downs, and wages were then paid only in company scrip. "Wages— surprise!—were never quite enough to pay the bills. According to new laws that might or might not exist, people were not permitted to leave an employer to whom they owed money. They were obligated to work off the debt either as quasi-indentured people or as convicts. That is, if they refused to work, they could be arrested, jailed, and in the end, handed over to their employers" (*Sower*, 259). Thus, "debt slavery" is made an institution. A law exists that forces adults—or their children—to work off unavoidable debt.

Medical care for people in such abysmal circumstances is nonexistent. There are no doctors, and no one can afford over-the-counter medications, so they use herbs grown in tiny gardens instead. Emery's husband had died on the dirt floor of their shack without ever seeing a doctor for what sounds to Bankole like peritonitis brought on by untreated appendicitis. "Such a simple thing. But then, there's nothing more replaceable than unskilled labor" (*Sower*, 259). Emery eventually runs away from the group, and a twosome joins them, Grayson and Doe Mora, who "both show the tendency to drop to the ground and roll into a fetal knot when frightened" (*Sower*, 262), suggesting to Lauren that they had formerly been slaves. Knowing the further possibilities for slavery in the current economic and political climate, Lauren characterizes her group as "the crew of a modern underground railroad," helping former slaves—contemporary slaves in an economy that had arrived even sooner than she and her father had thought it would. "My god," says Bankole, "this country has slipped back 200 years" (*Sower*, 274).

One of the technological innovations in literal slavery is the invention of the collar, a device that permits absolute control of the wearer. At any deviation from the owner's instructions, the wearer is subjected to excruciating electrical pain or choking. Sex slaves are collared, as are prisoners or any human—adult or child—who is captured and sold to the highest bidder. As Lauren's brother Marcus, who was collared for years, tells her, the worst thing is that "most people don't die of it" (*Sower*, 130).

Bankole eventually tells Lauren that he owns 300 heavily wooded (and potentially safe) acres farther north with wells for water, and he asks her to marry him. Lauren agrees only on the condition that the whole group can join them. Bankole, Lauren, and their companions move forward with uncertainty and tenuous hope. They are, as Lauren says, "a harvest of survivors" (*Sower*, 265). All of the members of Earthseed must learn what it means to survive, however—that it means more than merely staying alive. When Allie's sister, Jill, is killed, Lauren helps her grieve and gives her the message, "*In spite of your loss and pain, you aren't alone. You still have people who care about you and want you to be all right. You still have family*" (*Sower*, 272; emphasis in original). A radical statement in a time of such scarcity and nearly unimaginable brutality, Lauren's vision of community holds throughout the group's ordeal.

Despite Bankole's assurances that the land is safe and suitable for "farming . . . and logging, and just plain isolated living" (*Sower*, 281), they find only the bones and ashes of his sister and her family and the remains of the house. They realize that no place is invulnerable but decide to remain anyway and attempt to build a community of survival. They have learned difficult lessons from their peregrinations on the road: that living as loners is perilous if not futile, acknowledging that two adults alone could not have kept a good watch, but that with their numbers, they might be able to do better. Bankole and Lauren understand that as bad as things are in the society, "we haven't even hit bottom yet. Starvation, disease, drug damage, and mob rule have only begun. Federal, state, and local governments still exist—in name at least—and sometimes they manage to do something more than collect taxes and send in the military" (*Sower*, 295). For obvious reasons, the seekers decide to name the community Acorn, and the book ends with the hopeful passage from Luke 8:5–8, the parable of the sower and the seed that was sown on good ground.

Talents begins in 2090, as Lauren and Bankole's adult daughter, Larkin (or Asha Vere, as she has been named by her Christian America foster parents), is reading her mother's journals and the few papers left by her father. She looks back over the crisis-ridden and chaotic historical moment known as the Apocalypse, or more popularly ("more bitterly," writes Bankole), the "Pox." Although historical record marks the period from 2015 until 2030, Bankole argues that it began well before 2015, perhaps at the turn of the millennium, and probably still has not ended even by 2032 (*Talents*, 13).

> I have also read that the Pox was caused by accidentally co-
> inciding climatic, economic, and sociological crises. It
> would be more honest to say that the Pox was caused by
> our own refusal to deal with obvious problems in those
> areas. We caused the problems: then we sat and watched as
> they grew into crises. . . . I have seen enough to know that
> it is true. I have watched education become more a privi-
> lege of the rich than the basic necessity that it must be if
> civilized society is to survive. I have watched as conve-
> nience, profit, and inertia excused greater and more dan-
> gerous environmental degradation. I have watched poverty,
> hunger, and disease become inevitable for more and more
> people. [*Talents*, 14]

Physicians are scarce during the Pox and its repressive aftermath. For example, Halstead, a community that tried to hire Bankole, is finally able to bring a young physician whom no one trusts simply because of his age; no one believes he is a real doctor, since "these days, almost all young physicians—those under 50—were working in privatized or foreign-owned cities, towns, or huge farms. There, they could earn enough to give their families good lives and the company police would keep them safe from marauding thugs or desperate poor people. There had to be something wrong with a 35-year-old doctor who was still looking for a place to hang out his shingle" (*Talents*, 160). Butler underscores medicine's vulnerabilities by linking disease, illness, and injury with the social conditions that inertia and profit have allowed to run rampant. In this critical dystopian scenario, all young doctors have had to sell themselves to "owned" cities, towns, or farms in order to be protected and to obtain any measure of quality of life. The choice is not so far off the kinds of choices medical students face when looking at the huge debts accrued in school vis-à-vis the kinds of salaries and lifestyles offered by the urgent, difficult practice of medicine in urban or rural poor areas, for example.

Acorn's success is problematic. The community thrives and makes a living by farming and light hauling. Under the repressive Christian America government, which was voted into place as a response to the earlier chaos and violence, all who do not stand with the president and his conservative civic gospel are suspect and vulnerable (reminding one of George W. Bush's chilling announcement shortly after September 11, 2001, that one would be either "for" or "against" the United States in its fight against "terrorism"). Civil liberties are nonexistent. Christian America's Crusaders mean to crush all "cults" that do not preach and live by the Christian America gospel. One day the Crusaders surprise Acorn (which has grown substantially) with their "maggots," huge tanklike devices that are impervious to bullets, bombs, fire, or any other weaponry. They paralyze the people with a poison gas, which kills several, including Bankole (because of his age) and Zarah, who is small. Once Acorn is subdued and captured, the women and men are separated and the children are sent to "decent, Christian" homes. Everyone is collared as a slave: "Once you've got a collar on, you can't run. Get a certain distance from the control unit and the collar chokes you. . . . Touch the control unit and the collar chokes you. It won't work for you anyway. It's got a fingerprint lock. . . . And of course, if you try to cut, burn, or otherwise damage the collar, it chokes you" (*Talents*, 120, 121). The men controlling the collars are able to restrain the wearer by emitting jolts of pain strong enough to cause unconsciousness. They can also manipulate neurological function to stimulate endorphins and produce a pleasure response, creating a dependency (needing the pleasure, fearing the pain) that drives some to suicide. Acorn is renamed a Christian Reeducation Camp (otherwise known as Camp Christian). Acorn members watch and listen carefully over the long, horrible months of their captivity, however, and when a violent storm and mudslide destroy the house in which the control unit for the slave collars is located, they murder their captors, release themselves, and flee.

The connection between the enslavement of this multiethnic community and the bondage of Africans in the United States is clear both in the treatment Acorn (and thousands of groups like it) receives and in the strategies of resistance the community uses. The difference is that in 2032 the discourse has changed. All are workers—slaves on a Christian plantation. The enslavement is a strategy of social control and containment of difference, however, rather than a means of economic empowerment (as it was in the white American South). Those who have not declared allegiance to the gospel of Christian America are suspect and vulnerable to being rounded up. "We must accept Jesus Christ as our Savior, Jarret's [the U.S. president] Crusaders as our teachers, Jarret as God's chosen restorer of America's greatness, and the Church of Christian America as our church. Only then will we be Christian patriots worthy to raise children" (*Talents*, 189), writes Lauren. It is no surprise that Jarret's Crusaders (they call themselves teachers), while exhorting them to "behave like decent Christian women" (*Talents*, 184), also regularly rape and beat them.

More quietly, the church and government of Christian America round up men accused of robbery, especially African American men (who are immediately thrown into jail and indentured to work for thirty days for the church). They are given a physical exam and required to donate blood at least twice. Lauren's friend, Day Turner, describes the offer made to him: "He had been encouraged . . . to donate a kidney or a cornea, after which he could heal and go free. . . . He refused, but he couldn't help knowing that his organs, and, in fact, his life could be taken from him at any time. Who would know? Who would care? He wondered why they had not already killed him" (*Talents,* 209). Sounding much like Trigg's schemes in *Almanac,* the church helps with the shortage of organs, again looking to the disposable population for harvestable commodities.

Throughout *Talents,* various characters captured in the camps question how the rest of the world (or country) can know what is going on in the "reeducation" camps and not do something about it. In *Talents,* Lauren asks, "How many people, I wonder, can be penned up and tormented—reeducated— before it begins to matter to the majority of Americans? How does this penning people up look to other countries? Do they know? Would they care?" (210). Many prisoners in the United States today ask questions along those same lines. Further, this is relevant to medicine because of the issue of community accountability: How can medicine do healing work when the nonmedical community is indifferent to (or ignorant of) social conditions causing both small and large medical catastrophes? Lauren conjectures that in the case of the church's indentured servitude program for accused (not yet convicted) robbers and others, "people with legal residences would be glad to see a church taking charge of the thieving, drug-taking, drug-selling, disease-spreading, homeless free poor" (*Talents,* 209). In other words, as long as they are out of sight, they are out of mind. Without advocacy and education, and without getting the attention of those who are comfortable, indifference stands as the norm. Thus the environment for abuse and oppression flourishes, and the disposable population of human beings grows, much as we see happening in U.S. jails and prisons today.

Acorn and those formerly imprisoned at Camp Christian know this well. Once they seize the opportunity and liberate themselves, they understand they must break apart in order to survive. They move in small teams or, in some cases, take up with people they meet on the highways. Everyone searches for their children or lost family members. They establish a place for message drops and spend months and years dispersed. Lauren continues to recruit followers for Earthseed. By the end of *Talents*, Jarret and Christian America have lost power and Earthseed has become quite large. Lauren finds her daughter, Larkin, although the reunion is difficult and Larkin never accepts her mother or Earthseed ("her other child, her older and best beloved child," Larkin bitterly laments). But Lauren's vision has borne fruit out of the "modelessness"; from the struggle of liminal unknowing a kind of *communitas* has occurred, and something new has been born.

> [Earthseed now] financed scientific exploration and in-
> quiry, and technological creativity. It set up grade schools
> and eventually colleges, and offered full scholarships to
> poor but gifted students. The students who accepted had to
> agree to spend seven years teaching, practicing medicine,
> or otherwise using their skills to improve life in the many
> Earthseed communities. Ultimately, the intent was to help
> the communities to launch themselves toward the stars
> and to live on the distant worlds they found circling those
> stars. [*Talents*, 340]

Earthseed is now wealthy and owns land, schools, farms, factories, stores, banks, and towns, and it has many well-known people among its ranks. Like the phoenix, Earthseed has risen from the ashes, and just before Lauren's death (at eighty-one), it launches its first shuttle of human cargo to Earth's first starship, the *Christopher Columbus*. ("I object to the name," says Lauren. "It's not about snatching up slaves and gold and presenting them to some European monarch. But one can't win every battle" [*Talents*, 363].)[21]

In addition, Lauren laments that things on Earth seem never to change:

We learn more and more about the physical universe, more about our own bodies, more technology, but somehow, down through history, we go on building empires of one kind or another, then destroying them in one way or another. We go on having stupid wars . . . but in the end, all they do is kill huge numbers of people, maim others, impoverish still more, spread disease and hunger, and set the stage for the next war. We can choose: We can go on building and destroying until we either destroy ourselves or destroy the ability of our world to sustain us. Or we can make something more of ourselves. We can grow up. [*Talents*, 321]

The community Lauren and her small band of followers will create is vulnerable and fragile, but it is community and not individualism that ultimately makes survival possible. These two novels and, indeed, all the novels discussed in this book call medicine into a renewed sense of community with the people who are most removed from it: the historically and socially marginalized. Butler challenges medicine to reconceptualize its role within the nonmedical community, to configure a new understanding of its relationship with and accountability to the broader community. The novels argue, in different ways, that this relationship must be one of mutual learning in different spaces. Madhu Dubey, discussing *Sower*, might well be talking about medicine when she says that the novel reveals "the impossibility of maintaining 'village' ideals of bounded community rooted in a stable locale" and that "the novel presents community as *process* rather than settlement."[22] For medicine, community as process occurs when a physician or health care practitioner allows her- or himself to move through unknowing into the radical space of *communitas* with patients and with members of the patient's community. Institutionally, it occurs when medical schools open their doors to alternative ways of thinking about illness and disease, and when hospitals and medical practitioners ask patients what they know about their illness and what other ways of healing they might pursue. It occurs every time a health care practitioner allows her- or himself to be a learner in spaces where medical training does not always go. It also occurs when hospitals and medical practices reach beyond the expertise contained within their own confines and ask the nonmedical community how best it may be served. This is a big order and one that the institution may never fill. But what if we envision medicine as being in process? Surely the shift from private practice to managed care has been a transformative journey for medicine, albeit a mostly negatively transforming one for physicians and patients alike. How might medicine resist dehumanizing trends?

As Lauren and the Earthseed community discover, existing in an individualistic mode is all but impossible in a brutal and imploding world. When Bankole predicts that the United States may "just break up into a lot of little states quarreling and fighting with each other over whatever crumbs are left," he criticizes the reification of borders, an issue taken up in Silko's *Almanac,* among others. This critique works in at least two ways. First, literally: violently enforcing borders—arbitrarily created systems of marking otherness—between countries, states, cities, and institutions is futile at best and self-destructive at worst. Second, on an individual level: sealing oneself off, imagining oneself as a unitary, self-sufficient autonomous subject, is again futile and ultimately destructive. By extension, medicine's tendency to stand alone within communities and the extraordinary diversity that comprises the United States, especially in urban areas but throughout the country as well, is to render itself vulnerable. Butler's novels challenge medicine to push forward, to make the connections between patients and social conditions, but to go even further, to enter its own journey through unknowing and into the myriad possibilities of *communitas.*

Coda
Trenchant Hope

In sickness are the stories of a broken world.
—Linda Hogan, "Sickness"

I promised to show you a map you say but this is a mural
then yes let it be   these are small distinctions
where do we see it from are the questions.
—Adrienne Rich, "An Atlas of the Difficult World"

The authors of the novels I have examined in this study construct representations of illnesses rooted in such social factors as racism, classism, sexism, domestic and sexual violence, and homophobia, as well as corruption and greed and other factors that contribute to the creation of the kind of infecting world that renders medicine itself vulnerable. From Velma Henry's apocalyptic visions in *The Salt Eaters* to Pecola Breedlove's terrible pain in *The Bluest Eye* to the reign of "Death-Eye Dog" in *Almanac of the Dead* and the horrible years of the Pox in *Parable of the Sower* and *Parable of the Talents*, these texts challenge the medical and nonmedical community alike. I have read the novels for their critiques as well as for what I think of as "roads to the possible." Those roads are difficult and not clearly drawn. As Adrienne Rich writes, we may end up with textual murals rather than tidy maps. These murals/maps provide constructions of sick bodies that cannot be separated from sick social worlds, insisting over and over that the idea of health localized in individual bodies is a myth. But the novels also call for a paradoxical recognition of medicine's limits and, at the same time, a willingness to transgress its boundaries and join forces with the nonmedical community to work for social change as well as to understand and embrace alternatives to biomedical care when appropriate.

A few years ago I studied a thick medical chart with an interdisciplinary group of colleagues—another literary scholar, a communications scholar, and a physician. We asked what reading this chart as a literary text would tell us about what appeared to have been a particularly difficult series of encounters. The chart narrated a fractured story of one women's frustrating battle to ease chronic pain through a total of sixty-nine visits in six years with no relief at all. In the entire chart, we found no record of anyone having suggested that the patient try alternatives to standard biomedical treatment. We saw no consulting beyond the boundaries of biomedicine. The chart told its own story of medicine's continued sense of itself as the final word. Indeed, as it became increasingly clear that standard medical treatments were not working, the discourse of the chart subtly began to shift in tone, blaming the *patient* for her pain—her probable neuroses or, as one chart writer suggested, the possibility that she was simply a malingerer. Operating as an institutional loner, isolated from other healing alternatives, medicine had unnecessarily failed this patient.[1] Recognizing limitations suggests calling on other resources, indeed, having knowledge of other resources. But another issue the novels in this study raise over and over is the interconnection between sick bodies and a sick world. The narratives break down strict binary oppositions, insisting that a patient is always already part of a larger social context; healing of individuals will come about only with concomitant social change.

Jonathan Mann, in looking at medicine, public health, ethics, and human rights, underscores the obvious—that social factors are major determinants of health throughout the world (the rich live longer, healthier lives)—and he grapples with the question of physicians' roles in human rights.[2] He equates the use of ethics primarily with medicine (and its concern with individuals) and human rights with public health (and its concern with populations), but he questions such strict demarcations and calls for bridges between the two fields. He asks how a human rights perspective might be relevant to individual medical practitioners. Such a perspective clearly goes beyond the necessarily limited medical view. Mann provides the example of a woman being treated in an emergency room with injuries inflicted by her spouse and asks, "To what extent is the physician responsible for ensuring access to care for marginalized populations in the community, or helping the community understand the medical implications of public policy measures, or identifying, responding to and preventing discrimination occurring within medical institutions?" He continues, "Where, that is, does the boundary of medicine end?" Rather than answering the question, he leaves it for further ethical discussion, "at the frontiers of human rights and public health."[3]

Feminists such as Evelyn C. White, Dorothy E. Roberts, Carole Warshaw, and Susan Sherwin and scholars such as Howard Waitzkin argue that it is indeed the responsibility of medicine to narrow the gap between individual and social issues.[4] Additionally, however, the nonmedical community also must be an integral part of and have accountability in puzzling out various ways to deal with these issues. All of the novels in this study push medicine to think of itself as part of a broad system of public health, to focus on collectivities. But if resources within the nonmedical community are not available (or are invisible) to deal with social problems, or if the divide between nonmedical and medical resources remains, much is wasted; little can be done.

This is not to let medicine off the hook. Countless times as I have been working on this project, I have imagined physicians reading over my shoulder, rolling their eyes, telling me to get real. But what I know when I stop to think about it is that the imaginary physicians are quite different from many of the real clinicians in my life—those whose patient I am and those with whom I am a friend or colleague. Those who work part time in private practice to support themselves so that they can spend time practicing or teaching at Cook County Hospital, those who speak out against military occupation in Palestine or against police brutality here in the United States, those who refuse to let hospitals overlook battered women, those who are working in El Salvador among rural poor people, those who struggle to bring AIDS care to impoverished communities, those who quietly ask their patients in urban or rural offices what else might be bringing them in besides their cough or what other questions they might have or what life at home is like, or those who join hands with neighborhood partners to create health programs such as Westside Chicago's Mile Square or the Chicago Women's Health Center—those practitioners offer the possibility that medicine can change. But they are only individual examples.

The novelists in this study offer what I would like to call trenchant hope for medicine and society. In the construction of characters and societies in which medicine's failings as well as its possibilities emerge, they invite readers to pay attention; to look carefully at our world, our communities, and how we live; and in that looking, to think about medicine and its relationship to illness and health. In their sometimes direct, sometimes oblique ways, the novels push medicine to shift its sights from illness as an individual condition confined to individual bodies and to look instead at the murky, messy, but powerful politics of medicine, calling for the complex process of individual, institutional, and social change. This is no small order, but it is one that each of the texts, in manifold ways, insists we are capable of. Together.

Notes

Introduction

1. Capacitar exists in Suchitoto because of the wisdom and endurance of the Salvadoran women themselves. It is also due in part to the work of Sr. Pat Farrell, who lived in the region throughout the war and who brought Patricia Cane, Ph.D., to the area to train many of the religious workers there. More important, however, they have taught the Salvadoran women to train one another and to provide leadership in surrounding pueblos in promoting the health of women damaged by trauma. For more on Capacitar's beginnings, see Cane's website, www.capacitar.org. Also see Stanford, "Women's Advocacy and Healing."

2. George Engel first used the term "biopsychosocial" in 1977 and 1978. Much writing about medicine today relies on an understanding of the shift Engel's model necessitates.

3. Davis, "Sick and Tired of Being Sick and Tired," 19. In this article Davis notes that "Afro-American women are twice as likely as white women to die of hypertensive cardiovascular disease, and they have three times the rate of high blood pressure. Black infant mortality is twice that of whites, and maternal mortality is three times as high. Lupus is three times more common among Black women than white, thus the funds channeled into research to discover a cure for it have been extremely sparse. Black women die far more often than white women from diabetes and cancer" (ibid., 21). Laurie Kaye Abraham's *Mama Might Be Better Off Dead* also highlights graphically the plight of poor African American women—indeed all urban poor women—in the United States who face a health care system that is incapable of dealing with the complexities of life on the fringes of society.

4. Henderson et al., *Social Medicine Reader*, 3.

5. This observation does not belong solely to the domain of feminist thought, however. Much work in medical anthropology and sociology as well as in literature and medicine addresses these issues from a variety of perspectives. As Virginia Warren says, new and important directions for medical ethics quite possibly draw on ideas from Marxism or the holistic health movement; see Warren, "Feminist Directions." A feminist perspective will inform medical ethics, possibly change it, but it will not be the only informing and changing agent.

6. Sherwin, *No Longer Patient*, 6.

7. Ibid., 84.

8. Warren, "Feminist Directions," 32.

9. Ibid., 35.

10. Waitzkin, *Politics of Medical Encounters*. Waitzkin uses the example of a woman with heart irregularities that are interfering with her ability to do housework. "The doctor checks an electrocardiogram while she exercises, changes her cardiac medications, and congratulates her in her efforts to maintain a tidy household" (ibid., 3).

11. Ibid., 23.

12. Ibid., 11.

13. Farmer, "Listening for Prophetic Voices."

14. Taussig, "Reification," 3.

15. I am indebted to former and present members of the Chicago Narrative Group for creative and challenging discussions of the work of Sherwin, Waitzkin, and Taussig, especially Kathryn Montgomery, Suzanne Poirier, Barbara F. Sharf, Daniel Brauner, and William Donnelly.

16. Simon and Manier, "Ravenswood Hospital."

17. Tanner, "Teen Dies Near Hospital."

18. Ad Hoc Committee to Defend Health Care, "For Our Patients, Not for Profits," 436. The authors note that the profits per day per patient for hospital chains reach $100 and that a takeover deal of a health maintenance organization nets $990 million. In addition, insurers' overhead consumes $46 billion annually.

19. See, e.g., Montello, "Narrative Competence," 186, which states that "applying a narrative approach to ethical problems reframes the issues by focusing attention on the context of a patient's and family's life in all its moral complexity." Also see Hilde Lindemann Nelson, *Stories and their Limits*, and Anne Hudson Jones, "Darren's Case."

20. Brody, "Who Gets to Tell the Story?," 29.

21. Sayles interview.

22. Gay Wilentz, in *Healing Narratives*, looks at African-based healings in Erna Brodber's *Jane and Louisa Will Soon Come Home* and Toni Cade Bambara's *Salt Eaters*. She also examines indigenous curative methods in Leslie Marmon Silko's *Ceremony* and Keri Hulme's *Bone People*. Also see Wilentz, *Binding Cultures*.

23. Gayl Jones's *Song for Anninho* (1999) has just been reprinted. See also her *Corregidora*, *Eva's Man*, and *The Healing*. All of these texts deal with illness and healing and the complicated social contexts from which they arise. Walker's *Possessing the Secret of Joy*, *Color Purple*, *Temple of My Familiar*, and *Meridian* could also have been included, among a host of others. Ntozake Shange's choreopoem, *for colored girls who have considered suicide/when the rainbow is enuf*, is a text in which the ensemble cast moves from individual pain to a communal affirmation of the possibility of wholeness and healing. Also see Marita Bonner's "Drab Rambles," in *Frye Street and Environs*. Obviously there are also white women writing about issues that challenge and help us redefine health and illness, Margaret Atwood being a good example. See especially her *Bodily Harm* and *Handmaid's Tale*.

24. Roberts, "Reconstructing the Patient," 116–17.

25. Bellah et al., *Habits of the Heart*, 153.
26. Ibid.

Chapter 1

This chapter was first published in shorter form as "Mechanisms of Disease" in the *NWSA Journal* 6.1 (1994): 28–47, and I am grateful to Gay Wilentz for her helpful comments on an initial draft. I am also indebted to Trudier Harris for her interest and support in the very nascent stages of this chapter.

1. All quotations from Bambara, *Salt Eaters*; Paule Marshall, *Praisesong for the Widow*; and Naylor, *Women of Brewster Place*, will be cited parenthetically within the text.

2. Some consensus has been reached on the distinctions between terms such as "illness," "disease," and "sickness." Arthur Kleinman suggests that the experience of illness is culturally shaped and that "illness complaints are what patients and their families bring the practitioner," as opposed to disease, which "is what the practitioner creates in the recasting of illness in terms of theories of disorder" (Kleinman, *Illness Narratives*, 5). It is then that the patient's story is the illness and the doctor's is the disease, in Kleinman's formulation. Sickness, according to Kleinman, is "the understanding of a disorder in its generic sense across a population in relation to macrosocial (economic, political, institutional) forces" (ibid., 6). Sickness would be, in Kleinman's schema, the web of psychological and social factors that further compromise the illness experience. See also Brody's discussion of the terms in *Stories of Sickness*, esp. p. 21 n. 3. In this study, however, I use the terms "illness" and "sickness" interchangeably to denote the experience from the character's point of view as well as the network of forces that create, support, or maintain particular physical and mental symptoms. Of course, in using "illness" and "sickness" to mark social problems, I make a detour around medical paradigms and nosologies, attempting not to construct a diagnosis for the world but to use such terms as descriptive markers.

3. Maya Angelou's vignette in her well-known autobiography *I Know Why the Caged Bird Sings* underscores the access issue when the white (and only) dentist in town refuses to treat her painfully swollen jaw and infected tooth, saying "I'd rather stick my hand in a dog's mouth than in a nigger's" (160). See also Alice Walker's short story "Strong Horse Tea," in which the gap between Rannie Toomer and the white medical establishment she trusts absolutely is so wide, her child dies waiting for a doctor to whom Rannie's message of need is never even delivered.

4. I am thinking here of a well-known representation of African American culture and its contact with medicine. Ralph Ellison's hero in *Invisible Man* is virtually held hostage at a factory hospital, undergoing shock treatments until he has managed to convince the doctors that he can no longer remember his name, his mother's name, or who the African American trickster, Brer Rabbit, is; see *Invisible Man*, 231–45. See also Ellison's "Out of the Hospital and under the Bar" for an earlier (and quite different) version of this incident. Getting "well," in this case, requires no less than a complete

obliteration of history, culture, traditions, and identity. *Invisible Man* seems to reverse paradigms such as Howard Brody's, which argues that to be ill is to have one's identity altered (*Stories of Sickness*). Here the main character is pronounced "well" or cured only when he seems to have *accepted* an altered, less African, identity—an identity enforced and reinforced by the medical establishment itself. (Of course, the character "changes the joke and slips the yoke," as Ellison would say, simply appearing to comply as a means to escape the racist and immoral medical treatment to which he is subject.)

5. Traylor, "Music as Theme," 63.

6. Sherwin, *No Longer Patient*, 156.

7. Hoagland, *Lesbian Ethics*, 145.

8. Bellah et al., *Habits of the Heart*, 143.

9. Similarly, Alice Walker's *Meridian* connects racism and social injustice with her character Meridian's own unnamed illness, which, among other things, renders her prostrate and eventually causes her to lose her hair. Somewhat like Velma, Meridian is a revolutionary who has "remain[ed] close to the people" but who succumbs to an enervating physical condition, the recovery from which involves picking up lost pieces of her past and becoming once again ready to "go back to the people, live among them, like Civil Rights workers used to do" (ibid., 31).

10. Brown, "Afro-Caribbean Spirituality." Similarly Bambara, discussing her work as a writer, asks, "Is it natural (sane, healthy, whole-some, in our interest) to violate the contracts/covenants we have with our ancestors, each other, our children, ourselves, and God? . . . In *Salt* . . . the question is, do we intend to have a future as sane, whole, governing people?" ("Salvation Is the Issue," 47).

11. Holloway, *Moorings and Metaphors*, 119.

12. Busia, "What Is Your Nation?," 197.

13. Harris, "From Exile to Asylum," 157.

14. Great-aunt Cuney regularly tells Avey ("Avatara") the story of the African slaves at the Ibo Landing. When they were taken out of their boats, the Ibos looked around and saw "things that day you and me don't have the power to see" (*Praisesong*, 37), the slavery, the war, emancipation, and "everything after that right on up to the hard times today" (ibid., 38). With that the captive Africans, still chained, turned and walked singing right over the water "like [it] was solid ground" (ibid., 39) and headed home.

15. Wilentz, *Binding Cultures*, 111.

16. Wilentz points out African American and African women's "role in orally transmitting the values and mores of their culture" (ibid., xx), something she calls a " 'mothering' process of generational and cultural continuity" (ibid., xxi). The island women, surrounding and encouraging Avey as she rids her body of its poisons, in a sense "mother" Avey into a new conception of herself and her culture, much as the women in *Salt Eaters* and Mattie Michael in *Women of Brewster Place* do.

17. For a more extended discussion of Avey's "middle passage," see Busia, "What Is Your Nation?," 206–7, and Wilentz, *Binding Cultures*, 107.

18.   I am not suggesting here that the novel criticizes material gain as such. However, what is destructive is a materialism that becomes the end and goal of a life, and one defined by a white culture far removed from (and hostile to) the traditions and values of one's own culture and traditions.

19.   This passage brings to mind Zora Neale Hurston's description of the "Balm Yards" in Jamaica where healing baths are ritually given to people by operators who "are to their followers both doctor and priest" (*Tell My Horse*, 15).

20.   Karla Holloway notes similar imagery in *The Salt Eaters* where Velma becomes aware of "silvery tendrils . . . extending out like tiny webs of invisible thread . . . from her to Minnie Ransom to faintly outlined witnesses by the windows" (267). Holloway says that "Velma . . . is woven into a tapestry similar to the one Paule Marshall weaves in order to moor Avatara's lost spirit" (*Moorings and Metaphors*, 119).

21.   McClusky, "And Called Every Generation Blessed," 333.

22.   Christian, "Gloria Naylor's Geography," 355.

23.   Scarry, *Body in Pain*, 35.

24.   I am reminded of one of Frida Kahlo's well-known self-portraits, "The Broken Column," where the subject's body is represented by a segmented broken column girded with steel bands. In this painting, the female body does not simply "feel" pain but becomes a cage of pain, a prison, much as Ciel's body becomes a cage for her in Naylor's story.

25.   Trudier Harris has noted the strong connections between Minnie Ransom in *The Salt Eaters* and Mattie Michael. Both women use touch to connect and confront. She also notes that Ciel begins the healing process with vomiting ("getting the physical and emotional poison out of her system") much as Velma begins her journey out of darkness with grunts and growling; see "From Exile to Asylum," 163. In addition, however, Avey's vomiting and subsequent bath in *Praisesong for the Widow* have their corollary in *Brewster Place*. Michael Awkward describes Ciel's vomiting as a cleansing from the inside, her bath as a cleansing from the outside, and her tears as signifying the rejoining of Ciel's previously split selves; see "Authorial Dreams of Wholeness," 55.

26.   Certainly other sections of the novel address this issue as well. In "The Two," for example, violence and brutal rape are linked to homophobia, as well as to the constricted dreams and warped sense of manhood that infects C. C. and his gang.

27.   Waitzkin, *Politics of Medical Encounters*, 261.

28.   Sherwin, *No Longer Patient*, 238–39.

29.   See Roberts, "Reconstructing the Patient," 116–43.

Chapter 2

1.   All quotations from Silko, *Ceremony*, will be cited parenthetically in the text.

2.   Wald explains that "the difference between the cultural discrimination suffered by immigrant minorities and colonized minorities must be understood partly in terms of the degree of intensity of the discrimination and

partly in terms of the historical context in which the particular discriminatory act occurred." He warns readers against simplistic analyses and comparisons between colonized and immigrant groups, noting, as above, that the experiences are different and that not to recognize that is to treat those experiences reductively. See Wald, "Culture of 'Internal Colonialism,' " 21.

3.   Anzaldúa, *Haciendo Caras*, xix.

4.   Flores, "Claiming and Making," 53.

5.   Allen, *Sacred Hoop*, 62.

6.   hooks, "Narratives of Struggle," 57.

7.   Catherine Rainwater calls these "lyric chantways"; see her "Semiotics of Dwelling." Additionally, Ruppert, "Dialogism and Mediation," describes Silko's process as "mediation," where the two different spheres of discourse engage with each other and at the same time "express cross-cultural goals" (129). Ruppert says the poetry (or lyric chantways) "carry the traditional communal and mythic discourse of Laguna" (130).

8.   Slowik, "Henry James, Meet Spider Woman," 115.

9.   Silko uses the term "witchery" to denote an overarching evil that motivates human behavior and must be fought by way of retelling the story fashioned by the witches. In many ways, Silko's concept of witchery bears comparison with Judeo-Christian ideas as embodied by demons or the devil—an outside force that tempts and corrupts human existence. It is also important to note that many contemporary women's spirituality movements have embraced the concept of the "wicce" or witch as the embodiment of wisdom, a notion quite at odds with Silko's.

10.   Orr, "Theorizing the Earth," 147. For more on the significance of Ts'eh and female presence in the novel, see Antell, "Momaday, Welch, and Silko"; Swan, "Feminine Perspectives at Laguna Pueblo"; Allen, "Feminine Landscape"; and Flores, "Claiming and Making."

11.   I am not arguing here that war is restricted to the male domain. Jean Bethke Elshtain has demonstrated that for males to go to war, female complicity was necessary in creating a narrative of justification. The women functioned as "beautiful souls" to which the men would return, merging their warrior selves and being restored to a modicum of civility. See esp. Elshtain's chapter "Beautiful Souls, Just Warriors," in *Women and War*, 3– 13. My point is that the gender distinctions and roles themselves function as a system that makes war possible.

12.   hooks, "Narratives of Struggle," 54.

13.   Riley, "Mixed Blood Writer," 231.

14.   Anzaldúa, *Borderlands/La Frontera*, 3.

15.   For an extended discussion of Silko's (and Tayo's) mixed-blood heritage, see Riley, "Mixed Blood Writer."

16.   Ibid., 237.

17.   Flores says that "both the novel and the culture in which it is rooted are deeply committed to the conviction that story-telling is creation, in the most literal sense. . . . To tell a story is to make a reality; to act out a story is to make a world" ("Claiming and Making," 54).

18. It is not that genocide was not attempted in place of colonialism. The narrator of the novel points out that "White people selling Indians junk cars and trucks reminded Tayo of the Army captain in the 1860s who made a gift of wool blankets to the Apaches: the entire stack of blankets was infected with smallpox" (Silko, *Ceremony*, 158).

19. St. Andrews, "Healing the Witchery," 92, 90.

20. Crow Dog and Erdoes, *Lakota Woman*, 22; emphasis in original.

21. Ibid., 30.

22. Ibid., 31.

23. Rich, "If Not with Others, How?," 203.

24. Frank, *Wounded Storyteller*, 28.

25. Kleinman, "Pain and Resistance," 174.

26. Swartz, "Colonizing the Insane," 51. See also Vaughan, *Curing Their Ills*, 125.

27. St. Andrews argues that "Western doctors in the Army psychiatric unit correctly diagnose [Tayo] to be suffering from battle fatigue, malaria and hallucinations[, but the] . . . diagnosis is . . . stuck in the dualisms of Cartesian thought, while Amerindian thought is based on circularity and interconnectedness" ("Healing the Witchery," 89).

28. This also recalls Ken Kesey's Native American character in *One Flew over the Cuckoo's Nest*. Throughout his hospitalization the Chief feigns the inability to speak, fooling the doctors and other health care workers until his final escape from the insane institution that has held him captive.

29. Hurtado, "Strategic Suspensions," 382.

30. Scarberry, "Memory as Medicine," 21.

31. Swan, "Feminine Perspectives at Laguna Pueblo," 313.

32. See Gwendolyn Brooks's perceptive description of Annie Allen's lover, returned from war bereft of his uniform and the intensity and excitement that had made him feel manly and alive. Back in the United States, he is quickly reminded that he is a black man and that by shedding his uniform he also sheds his power. See *Annie Allen* (1994), 103.

33. Bird, "Towards a Decolonization," 8.

34. Fanon, *Wretched of the Earth*, 47; emphasis in original.

35. This recalls Gwendolyn Brooks's sonnet sequence "Gay Chaps at the Bar," in *A Street in Bronzeville*. One of the sonnets, "the soldiers had their orders but the negroes looked like men," addresses the ridiculousness of segregated coffins as the white soldier ponders the shared humanity among the different colors of dead soldiers.

36. Bevis, "Homing In," 582.

37. Swan describes Ts'eh: "Tayo quietly observes Ts'eh preparing her herbs and medicines, paraphernalia signaling her role as a medicine woman and rainmaker. She brings lifegiving moisture—the snow and rain . . . using her stormcloud blanket and crooked willow staff, and her potency is encoded in the eagle rainbirds imprinted on the silver buttons of her moccasins" ("Feminine Perspectives at Laguna Pueblo," 319–20).

38. Tayo's grandmother's blindness may have been exacerbated by the test explosion. While Tayo realizes where he stands, he remembers that Old Grandma had told him about something that happened in his absence: "There was a flash of light through the window. So big, so bright even my old clouded-up eyes could see it. It must have filled the whole southeast sky" (Silko, *Ceremony*, 245).

39. For more on the significance of this place, see Garcia, "Senses of Place"; Rainwater, "Semiotics of Dwelling"; Robert M. Nelson, "Place and Vision"; and Schweninger, "Writing Nature."

40. Women also felt the burden of reintegrating (white) male veterans into the workforce. The thousands of women who had been recruited or cajoled into working technical jobs during the war found themselves quickly edged out to make room for the white men returning home who would need immediate employment.

41. The book deals with many issues, among them the disposability of many veterans, especially those who are dark skinned, poor, and marginalized. Tayo's friends are at a loss as to what to do with their lives now that they are back on the reservation with so few options open to them.

42. Crow Dog and Erdoes, *Lakota Woman*, 48.

43. As many have pointed out, in Laguna and Navajo tradition, the achievement of balance is characteristic of healing, and illness signifies a lack of balance or harmony. Toni Flores notes that "in this world there is a proper order to the universe, an order that includes humans, sentient and nonsentient material beings, and spirits; all evil, illness, misery, and natural disasters result from a disruption of this proper order" ("Claiming and Making," 53–54).

44. Winsbro, *Supernatural Forces*, 184.

45. Kleinman, *Writing at the Margin*, 35–36.

Chapter 3

A somewhat abbreviated version of this chapter is forthcoming in Patricia Moran and Tamar Heller, *Scenes of the Apple: Food and the Female Body in Nineteenth and Twentieth Century Women's Writing*.

1. Titus, " 'This Poisonous System,' " 200.

2. Edwidge Danticat's novel *Breath, Eyes, Memory* is a notable departure from the usual connection of eating disorders with white middle-class women. In it the protagonist, a Haitian American, struggles with bulimia and the effort to come to terms with her sexuality, her family heritage, and her identity.

3. Becky W. Thompson, *A Hunger So Wide and So Deep*, 6.

4. See, e.g., Orbach, *Fat Is a Feminist Issue* and *Hunger Strike*; Chernin, *Obsession* and *Hungry Self*; Brumberg, *Fasting Girls*; Lelwica, *Starving for Salvation*; and Furst and Graham, *Disorderly Eaters*.

5. All quotations from Morrison, *Beloved*, will be cited parenthetically within the text.

6. Schapiro, "Bonds of Love," 198.

7. Berger, "Ghosts of Liberalism," 415.

8.   Bordo, *Unbearable Weight*, 11; emphasis in original.

9.   Becky W. Thompson, *A Hunger So Wide and So Deep*, 17.

10.   hooks, "Living to Love," 333.

11.   Ibid., 334.

12.   Henderson, "Re-Membering the Body as Historical Text," 79.

13.   Winsbro, *Supernatural Forces*, 130.

14.   Foucault, "Two Lectures," 98.

15.   Laub, "Bearing Witness," 62.

16.   Koolish, "Fictive Strategies," 425. Koolish also points out that the "extravagant feast" given by Sethe and Baby Suggs after Sethe's escape is "Sethe's failed attempt to provide a community stay against spiritual and physical hunger, metaphorically, to feed 'Sixty million and more,' to feed a hunger that spanned continents and time frames, to quench a thirst that the subsequently arriving Beloved will bring from another time, another place" (ibid.).

17.   Ibid., 426.

18.   Scheper-Hughes, *Death without Weeping*, 128.

19.   Handley, "House a Ghost Built," 699.

20.   Quotation in Fraden, *Imagining Medea*, 77.

Chapter 4

1.   See, for example, Williams and Williams-Morris, "Racism and Mental Health."

2.   See, for example, Rollock and Gordon, "Racism and Mental Health." They sketch out several "mechanisms of influence" that maintain and reproduce racism: definition (what behaviors are considered pathological); etiology (racist explanations of origins of mental disorders); evaluation (tools that have been developed by those in socially advantaged situations); service delivery (availability of "ethnoculturally diverse" service providers, attention to prevention, cultural appropriateness of major treatment models); institutional structure (systems often at variance with folkways and lifestyles of diverse population); research (open to racist assumptions, culture-bound epistemology and uses); and training (that fails to provide relevant direct service skills, to promote diverse research, or to encourage attention to oppressed contexts).

3.   Farmer, "On Suffering," 263.

4.   Peterson, "History, Postmodernism," 984. Peterson also points out that "European diseases such as smallpox, measles, and tuberculosis are said to have been more deadly to native populations across the country than Indian-white warfare was" (ibid., 985). She cites Carl Waldman's claim that disease wiped out 25 to 50 percent of Native Americans, while warfare killed an estimated 10 percent; see ibid., 992 n. 10.

5.   Christian, "Contemporary Fables," 60.

6.   Quoted in LeClair, "Language Must Not Sweat," 29.

7.   Yetman, *Majority and Minority*, 217.

8. Ibid., 221.

9. Ibid., 223.

10. Silko's *Ceremony* also figures the effects of internalized racism in terms of the mutilated, sick, and tortured body manifest in Rocky's injury and death, the torture and eventual death of Harley, and Tayo's own illness. The "witchery" manifests itself again and again, in Silko's universe, as that force of racism that operates both externally and internally to carry out a genocidal agenda.

11. Waitzkin, *Politics of Medical Encounters*.

12. Peterson, "History, Postmodernism," 990.

13. All quotations from Erdrich, *Tracks*, and Morrison, *Bluest Eye*, will be cited parenthetically within the text.

14. hooks, *Black Looks*, 191.

15. Susan Pérez Castillo, "Postmodernism," 293.

16. Ibid., 284.

17. Pauline's hatred of her daughter continues throughout her life. In Erdrich's *Love Medicine* we find out that the nearly fourteen-year-old Marie enters the Sacred Heart Convent for a time, wanting to be a saint "from this reservation" that the nuns would "have to kneel to" (43). The convent is a "catchall place for nuns that don't get along elsewhere. Nuns that complain too much or lose their mind" (ibid., 45). In what may be one of the most memorable novelistic mother-daughter relationships, Marie encounters the sadistic Sister Leopolda (her mother, Pauline Puyat), who pours scalding water on her back ("to warm your cold ash heart"), stabs her with a fork, and knocks her out with a fire poker. Hertha Wong argues that "both Marie and Leopolda must create an identity in isolation. Leopolda seeks escape in solitude and isolation, while Marie attempts to reconstruct family and community" (Wong, "Adoptive Mothers," 182).

18. Stoudt, "Medieval German Women."

19. Palmer, Sherrard, and Ware, *Philokalia*, 143.

20. Kavanaugh and Rodriguez, *Collected Works*, 204.

21. Morris, *Culture of Pain*, 135.

22. Wong, "Adoptive Mothers," 185.

23. Cassell, "Nature of Suffering."

24. Interestingly, the connection between the decision to amputate and a callous lack of concern for the patient is taken up in Melville's *White-Jacket*, where the power of medicine and the class status of the ailing sailor makes it possible for Dr. Cuticle to perform with impunity an amputation that kills the unfortunate (and low-ranking) sailor. Some hundred years later, Alan Gurganus takes up this theme in his novel *The Oldest Living Confederate Widow Tells All* but revises it. Here a wounded (and, once again, low-ranking) Civil War soldier is about to have his leg amputated by a rushed and uncaring surgeon. The leg is saved through the agency of a loyal (if slightly drunk) friend who forces the surgeon at gunpoint to operate (which he does successfully) rather than amputate.

25. Butler-Evans, *Race, Gender, and Desire*, 64, 66.

26.   Scarry, *Body in Pain*, 47.

27.   Many critics have argued that for Pauline the issue of displacement is at the root of her problems, that the urban North fails to give her the space for imagination and the landscape that would allow her to see beauty in terms of natural phenomena, not constructed ideals. See, for example, Christian, *Black Feminist Criticism*, 48.

28.   This brings to mind the ideological systems of the nineteenth century that considered white, upper-class women exquisitely sensitive to pain and the "heartier" Irish peasant stock to be much less so. Black women were thought to be nearly impervious, thus justifying all manner of abuses. See Pernick, *Calculus of Suffering*. More recently, studies of pain treatment have demonstrated that African Americans and other people of color are usually undertreated for pain, this time due in part to stereotypes of drug addiction. See, for example, Morrison et al., " 'We Don't Carry That' "; Todd et al., "Ethnicity and Analgesic Practice"; and Ng et al., "Ethnic Differences in Analgesic Consumption for Postoperative Pain" (interestingly, in this study the authors cannot determine whether the differences in analgesics used reflect patient behavior/attitudes or staff behavior/attitudes or both).

29.   Bennett, "Mother's Part," 132.

30.   Farmer, "On Suffering," 272.

31.   Ridley, Chih, and Olivera, "Training in Cultural Schemas."

32.   Hollar, "Impact of Racism."

Chapter 5

1.   Tjaden and Thoennes, "Prevalence, Incidence, and Consequences of Violence against Women."

2.   World Health Organization, Department of Injuries and Violence Prevention, http://www.who.int/violence—injury—prevention/vaw/infopack.htm. This website contains extensive materials and resources for anyone interested in domestic violence and health. It also has many suggestions for medicine's response to domestic violence.

3.   Warshaw, "Domestic Violence," 201.

4.   Herman, *Trauma and Recovery*, 3.

5.   Warshaw, "Domestic Violence," 202.

6.   Ibid. In another study, Warshaw analyzed fifty-two medical records of women who came into emergency rooms with physical trauma and found that in more than 90 percent of the cases, physicians "failed to obtain a psychosocial history, failed to ask about sexual abuse or a past history of physical abuse, failed to ask about the woman's living arrangements, and neglected to address the woman's safety." Furthermore, "in seventy-eight percent of the cases, the physician failed to identify the relationship of the assailant to the victim" (Warshaw, "Limitations of the Medical Model," 511).

7.   Warshaw, "Domestic Violence," 203.

8.   Ferraro, "Dance of Dependency," 77–78.

9.   Ibid., 77, 79.

10.   Heberle, "Deconstructive Strategies," 67.

11.   Ibid., 65.

12.   Ibid., 67.

13.   Of course there are many other texts I could have included in this chapter. I have chosen Cisneros, Campbell, and Sapphire because of the issues of silence and the birth of language, as well as the socioeconomic status of the characters and the complicated issues it raises. One notable novel is Patricia Chao's *Monkey King*. In it the main character, a highly educated Chinese American woman, the daughter of two professors, comes to terms with her father's sexual abuse by finding people in the family with whom to have her experiences validated and, most especially, through her work as a visual artist. Struggling with tendencies toward self-mutilation and a suicide attempt, through a great deal of therapy and her own soul-gathering process, Sally Wang is finally able to say, in the last line of the novel, both that "life is exquisite" and "I need all the luck I can get."

14.   Along with Chao's novel, another is Ann Patchett's *Magician's Assistant*, in which the son of a rural white family kills his father in defense of his mother, whom the father beats regularly.

15.   Herman, *Trauma and Recovery*, 8.

16.   Farmer, "On Suffering," 280.

17.   Scarry, *Body in Pain*, 35.

18.   Ibid., 6.

19.   The 1975 Declaration of Tokyo defines torture as "the deliberate, systematic or wanton infliction of physical or mental suffering by one or more persons, acting alone or on the orders of any authority, to force another person to yield information, to make a confession, or for any other reason" (www.wma.net/e/policy/17-f—e.html). While domestic violence is probably not carried out under orders, it certainly fits much of this definition. In no way, however, do I want to detract from the horror of state-authorized torture. Rather, I believe the similarities between the two are instructive and illustrative. I was interested to read Mary Fabri's broad definition of torture presented at the University of Chicago's Human Rights Program Conference on Torture: "the physical and psychological infliction of pain and anguish executed in a strategic fashion to punish, coerce, and/or control an individual and/or a group or community of which that individual is a member. This means that actual physical and/or psychological torture may be inflicted on one individual, but the impact profoundly affects the family, community and other significant affiliations that an individual has." (Fabri directs the Marjorie Kovler Center for the Treatment of Survivors of Torture.)

20.   Russo, *Taking Back Our Lives*, 186.

21.   All quotations from Cisneros, "Woman Hollering Creek," in *Woman Hollering Creek and Other Stories*, will be cited parenthetically in the text.

22.   A study of 400 undocumented women in the San Francisco Bay area in 1990 revealed that 34 percent had experienced some form of domestic violence; see Hogeland and Rosen, "Needs Assessment of Undocumented Women."

23. Doyle, "Haunting the Borderlands," 54. See also Mullen, "Silence between Us Like Language."

24. Cleófilas's fascination with romantic love in *telenovelas* and movies is not only like that of Pauline Breedlove in *The Bluest Eye*, who takes her education in the movies and learns self-hate as a result, but I am also reminded of Gwendolyn Brooks's character Annie Allen in her long poem "The Anniad." Annie Allen is so overtaken by the idea of romance that she becomes involved in a painful relationship that leaves her with several children, bereft and hopeless at the end.

25. For more on the origins of La Llorona, see Anzaldúa's *Borderlands/La Frontera* and Carbonell's "From Llorona to Gritona."

26. Anzaldúa, *Borderlands/La Frontera*, 33.

27. When Jean Cocteau was recovering from an opium addiction, he recorded the experience of withdrawal not only in words but in drawings as well. One of them, *Por la boca de su herida* [Through the mouth of his wound], depicts a naked man with his head thrown back (and thus, voiceless) so that only the neck and torso are showing. One arm, cut off just above the elbow, reaches skyward, as though in supplication. On his right side is a bleeding gash with lips, tongue, and teeth. The gash itself is a mouth speaking with a long line of blood. The wound is the speaker and its language is the body itself. Cocteau knew well the power of the body to speak what words cannot. For more on this and other of Cocteau's drawings, see Stanford, "From the Mouth of Her Wound."

28. Mullen, "Silence between Us Like Language," 12.

29. All quotations from Campbell, *Your Blues Ain't Like Mine*, will be cited parenthetically within the text.

30. While Campbell constructs several parallel and intersecting plots, in this discussion I focus primarily on the construction of domestic violence and its connection to class and racism.

31. Freire describes *conscientização* as "the deepening of the attitude of awareness characteristic of all emergence" (*Pedagogy*, 109).

32. Frank, *Wounded Storyteller*, 18.

33. All quotations from Sapphire, *Push*, will be cited parenthetically within the text.

34. Hurston, *Their Eyes Were Watching God*, 112–13.

35. Richie, *Compelled to Crime*, 2. While Richie's analysis looks at women who have become entrapped in the criminal justice system, I believe her analysis holds true for Pecola and Precious and how they are viewed by society and the institutions within which both find themselves.

36. This is not to say that Precious leaves rage behind, but that with self-love, her rage becomes clarifying, cleansing, and focused.

37. Pemberton, "Hunger for Language," 3.

38. Roberts, *Killing the Black Body*, 17. Roberts points to a 1990 study in which 78 percent of white Americans said they believed that blacks preferred to live on welfare.

39.   Like Precious, Walker's main character, Celie, through the writing of letters, also shifts from victimization to almost inchoate rage to language that allows her to name her reality, with the help of Shug, and to construct a new reality for herself, one that is strong enough and capacious enough to include forgiveness and the creation of an entirely new form of community.

40.   Clarke, "Identity of One's Own," 38.

41.   McLeer and Anwar, "Study of Women."

42.   Bell and Mosher, "(Re)fashioning Medicine's Response," 229.

43.   Warshaw, "Domestic Violence," 208.

Chapter 6

1.   Among other things, these novels disrupt tidy notions of a mind/body split. I am reminded of David Morris's insistence that "the rigid split between mental and physical pain is beginning to look like a gigantic cultural mistake, perhaps similar to the belief that the world was flat" (Morris, *Culture of Pain,* 12).

2.   Fanon, *Wretched of the Earth,* 210.

3.   Would I want my brain surgeon to be pondering the unknowability of human existence as she is cutting? Of course not. But neither would I want her to rely only on lab values, especially at the expense of knowing who the patient beneath the knife was.

4.   Frank, *Wounded Storyteller,* 10.

5.   Bakhtin, "Epic and Novel," 23.

6.   Notably absent from my discussion is Gayl Jones, another writer who takes the question of truth and epistemology to task through her healer, Harlan Jane Eagleton. Harlan Jane is surprised by her gift of healing ("the point of them spirit gifts, the point of them spirit gifts, is that I am just a ordinary woman" [*The Healing,* 34]) but travels throughout the country participating in healing services where no one can explain what happens: "I lay my hands on a young woman suffering from a skin rash and immediately her skin become smooth and clear as a baby's. A elderly woman suffers from a bone ailment that make her lower back painful. I lay my hands on and she straightens, healthy, then bends forward and touches her toes. A baby's got chronic earache; I kiss both its little ears and they's made whole again" (ibid.). Weaving themselves through the novel are the Turtle Woman stories told by Harlan Jane's grandmother, tales of magic and transformation. It is through these stories as well as the healings that the notion of truth is held up for examination: "She smiled like she knew that her tale was the true one, or that a tale could be true and not be a true tale—that perhaps her Turtle Woman stories were truer than any carnival tale" (ibid., 136).

7.   See, for example, Hunter, "Making a Case"; Brody, *Healer's Power;* Hilde Lindemann Nelson, *Stories and Their Limits;* Chambers, "From the Ethicist's Point of View"; Charon, "Narrative Contributions to Medical Ethics"; and Kleinman, *Illness Narratives.*

8.   See the June 1996 issue of the *Journal of Medicine and Philosophy,* esp. Clouser, "Philosophy, Literature, and Ethics," and Hawkins, "Literature,

Philosophy, and Medical Ethics," for a good sense of the debate around narrative ethics.

9.   See esp. Anne Hudson Jones, "Darren's Case."

10.   Hunter, "Narrative," 1791.

11.   Charon et al., "Literature and Ethical Medicine," 243–44.

12.   Anne Hudson Jones, "Darren's Case," 283.

13.   Hunter, "Narrative," 1792.

14.   Ana Castillo, *Massacre of the Dreamers*, 146.

15.   *The Complete Poems of Emily Dickinson*, ed. Thomas H. Johnson (Boston: Little, Brown, 1960), 506–7.

16.   See, for example, Storhoff, " 'Only Voice Is Your Own.' "

17.   For more on Naylor's critique of George's (and to some extent Cocoa's) appropriation of white values, see Meisenhelder, " 'Whole Picture' " (quotation on 405).

18.   Obviously these are not the only novels to treat alternative healing and uncertain etiologies. Cofer's *Line of the Sun* includes a character who is an herbalist (and who is both vilified by some in the community as a whore and revered by others as a healer). In the Introduction I mentioned Divakaruni's *Mistress of Spices*, whose central character heals through her use of spices (which she hears talking to her) and her ability to see into the hearts of her customers/patients. Of course, there is Gayl Jones's *The Healing*. Another less known but fascinating novel, Maria Thomas's *Antonia Saw the Oryx First*, deals with a physician (Antonia) who lives in East Africa and encounters Esther, a patient whose beliefs about her illness and injuries (there are reptiles living inside her) are directly counter to Antonia's (the pain is caused by a web of scar tissue and adhesions). Esther develops her own healing gifts that confound and illuminate Antonia's biomedical understanding and in part lead to her decision to return to the United States.

19.   Suzanne Poirier pointed out to me that while *Mama Day* is much less overtly Christian than *So Far from God*, Naylor's story itself is profoundly Christian in its themes of sacrifice and new life, while Castillo's novel, though interlaced with a syncretic blend of Latino Christianity, relies more on social, political, and folkloristic explanations for the kinds of illnesses and healings her characters experience.

20.   Storhoff, " 'Only Voice Is Your Own,' " 36.

21.   None of the characters in either novel and their methods of healing are without counterpart in the nonfictional world. To read Loudell Snow's accounts of healers in the African American community and their explanations is to recognize in them the various characters and events in *Mama Day*. For example, some of her chapter titles in *Walkin' over Medicine* sound as though they could have come right out of Miranda's mouth: "You'd Be Surprised What You Can Do with What You Have," "The Bible Says Watch as Well as Pray," "You Brought It on Your Own Self," "To Be Healthy You Must Have Good Blood," "God Doesn't Want Us to Misuse a Child—But He Wants Us to Be Firm." Similarly, the narratives in *Medicine Women, Curanderas, and Women Doctors*, especially those in the *curanderas* section,

resonate with the characters and events of *So Far from God*. There are interesting chapters on Sabinita Herrera, a *curandera* and *yerbera* (herbalist), and Jesusita Aragon, a *curandera* and *partera* (midwife), both of whom live in the Southwest and who sound a lot like Doña Felicia. Gregorita Rodriguez, a *curandera* and *sobardora* (who uses her hands to relieve abdominal symptoms) "relies faithfully on her own combination of factors—religion, *remedios*, and rubbing—to help her heal." She claims that "the doctors don't know anything about the stomach . . . and the curanderas know everything" (Perrone, Stockel, and Krueger, *Medicine Women, Curanderas, and Women Doctors*, 107, 108). Zora Neale Hurston, *Mules and Men*, 288–91, provides prescriptions from root doctors for gonorrhea, syphilis, bladder trouble, fistula, rheumatism, swelling, blindness, lockjaw, "flooding" (menstruation), nausea, "live things in stomach" (fits), "medicine to purge," "loss of mind" ("you drink some and give some to patient"), and "poisons."

22. All quotations from Naylor, *Mama Day*, and Ana Castillo, *So Far from God*, will be cited parenthetically in the text.

23. For more on Naylor's use of the quilt imagery, see Wagner-Martin, "Quilting," and Meisenhelder, " 'Whole Picture.' "

24. Tucker, "Recovering the Conjure Woman," 178.

25. Ibid., 179.

26. Latishia Simmons's description of healing powers resonates with similarity to Mama Day's methods:

> It's so many things we use! I don't know anything about *medicine*, real medicine, because you know this is all I was brought up with. Why, there's a lotta *weeds* out there *now*; why, you're walkin' over *medicine*! And greens we used, like dandelions. Dandelions is a *wonderful* food. There's so many vitamins out there right now that we're *walkin'* over. We walk *over* medicine, that's right. And the doctors say that people [who] wear copper bracelets for arthritis, that it's no *good* these days! I can't explain *what* it *was* about those remedies; it had to be some good because if it hadn't been some good they wouldn't have been able to provide. . . . And you'd be surprised what you can do with what you have. [Snow, *Walkin' over Medicine*, 34; emphasis in original].

27. Melzack and Wall, *Challenge of Pain*. The McGill-Melzack Pain Questionnaire asks sufferers to choose words in various groups, e.g., "flickering," "quivering," "pulsing," "throbbing," and "beating," in one category, and "punishing," "grueling," "cruel," "vicious," and "killing," in another (ibid., 62). See also their spatial display of pain descriptors on pp. 58–59.

28. In Naylor's next novel, *Bailey's Café*, it turns out that George's mother had been a pregnant fourteen-year-old Jew from Ethiopia, Mariam, who claims that she is a virgin; in fact, she is the Virgin Mary revisited. Given this genealogy, it makes sense that George's death becomes the life-giving salvation of Cocoa, cast as a Christ figure. Cocoa's illness—one that springs from an etiology of pure hatred and obsession—is only curable through love.

But George's perceptions of the truth of Cocoa's situation are so firmly embedded in his allegiance to the rational, explicable truth that he fails to keep his own life in saving Cocoa's. The novel does not make it clear that George needed to die for Cocoa, but that he instead needed to accept that her healing would not come through conventional means.

29.   Ana Castillo, *Massacre of the Dreamers*, 145, 154.

30.   Ibid., 153.

31.   In the same way, the methods of Franky's Tia Loretta and her prizewinning calabasas beg interpretation:

> "She injects them with Miracle-Gro, judge!" "She has a brujo come and do a ritual on her garden, judge! No normal calabasa could get that big!" They were very wrong, these poor excuses for gardeners and farmers, for Loretta's green thumb secret was as old as agriculture itself but had been forgotten so long that anyone knowing it would have suspected witchery, and that was that Loretta planted and harvested according to the *moon's* cycles, not the sun's. But how Loretta came upon this ancient wisdom is another secret, and yet another story. [Ana Castillo, *So Far from God*, 193; emphasis in original].

32.   Loca's sense of smell extends to the other world in the case of her father as well. When he returns after a twelve-year absence, she tells her mother that he has the smell of someone who has been in hell. " 'Only in hell do we learn to forgive and you got to die first,' La Loca said. 'That's when we get to pluck out all the devils from our hearts that were put there when we were *here*. That's where we get rid of all the lies told to us. That's where we go and cry like rain. Mom, hell is where you go to see yourself. This dad, out there, sitting watching T.V., he was in hell a long time. He's like an onion, we will never know all of him—but he ain't afraid no more' " (ibid., 42).

33.   Caridad predicts her sister Esperanza's journey to Saudi Arabia ("and she's afraid"), knowing that "no kind of white woman's self-help book and no matter how many rosaries she prayed, would result in giving her spirit the courage she got from the sweat lodge and which she surely needed now more than ever" (ibid., 47).

34.   "A medicine woman's power comes through her spirituality, evidenced in the healing ceremonies she performs. A *curandera's* power comes from her religion and her deep belief that God has selected her to heal on earth" (Perrone, Stockel, and Krueger, *Medicine Women, Curanderas, and Women Doctors*, 9).

35.   This is certainly true for Cocoa's illness, brought about by Ruby's intense jealousy, in *Mama Day*.

36.   In an interview, Native American medicine woman Dhyani Ywahoo offhandedly comments that her grandfather used to "put his hand in someone and take something out" in his curing ceremonies. See Perrone, Stockel, and Krueger, *Medicine Women, Curanderas, and Women Doctors*, 80.

37.   Frank, "Enacting Illness Stories," 41.

38. I am reminded of the chapel of the University of Central America José Simeón Cañas in San Salvador, El Salvador, where seven Jesuits and two women were brutally murdered in 1990 shortly before the twelve-year-long civil war ended. On the back wall of the chapel are fourteen large, framed, black-and-white drawings by Roberto Huezo of men and women being tortured or murdered, harsh expressions of naked violence. These are the university's stations of the cross and represent powerfully the Salvadoran people's understanding—like that of the women of Tome—of the seamless relevance of the torture and injustice of crucifixion and hope of resurrection to their own, daily, lived experience.

39. In Helena Maria Viramontes's wonderful and important novel, *Under the Feet of Jesus*, the character Alejo, a young farmworker, becomes mortally ill from exposure to crop dusters. (I also cannot resist mentioning her beautiful short story "The Moths," which incorporates elements of the inexplicable upon the death of a beloved grandmother. See *Moths and Other Stories*.)

40. Snow, *Walkin' over Medicine*, 43; emphasis in original. Even more challenging, perhaps, are the accounts of illness and disease that patients may (or more likely may not) bring into the clinical setting, accounts that rival those found in *Mama Day* and *So Far from God*.

> So this man, this other root man, just took a *hunch* of tellin' grandmother what to *do*, you know; what to *use*. And he gave my grandmother some kind of special *salve*. What it was I don't know; he gave her sumpin' to *rub* on it, keep puttin' on it, bathin' in it. And she did it. And sho 'nuff, right before everybody's eyes a snake crawled out of it . . . crawled outa that opening that was in her *leg*, crawl right clean outa there. And they killed it. They was hittin' at it and it just disappear, just like black magic, like voodoo or whatever. [Snow, *Walkin' over Medicine*, 5; emphasis in original].

41. Fadiman, *Spirit Catches You*, 261.

Chapter 7

I first presented several of the ideas in this chapter at the Annual Meeting of the Society for Health and Human Values in San Diego, California, October 1995. It was later published in slightly shorter form as " 'Human Debris': Border Politics, Body Parts, and the Reclamation of the Americas in Leslie Marmon Silko's *Almanac of the Dead*," in *Literature and Medicine* 16.1 (Spring 1997): 23–42.

1. For a discussion of the idea of social suffering, see Kleinman and Kleinman, "Appeal of Experience"; Das, "Language and Body"; Farmer, "On Suffering and Structural Violence"; and Lock, "Displacing Suffering," as well as the host of other fine articles contained in the *Daedalus* 125.1 (Winter 1996) issue.

2. Hearn, "Review," for example, hailed *Almanac* as a profound book of prophecy that draws on Silko's Native American heritage, feminism (this, I think, is highly debatable), and Marxism. Another critic calls it "one of the most ambitious literary undertakings of the past quarter century," albeit a

failed one; see Birkerts, "Apocalypse Now," 39. Niemann, in "New World Disorder," 1, claims that *Almanac* is the "best book" she has "read in years," one that is "an ark filled with the stories and the voices and the people who will create a new world out of the destruction of the old."

3. See Harjo, "World Is Round," 207–10; King, "New Epic for an Old World"; Coltelli, "Interview." (I want to thank A. LaVonne Ruoff for first alerting me to the King and Coltelli pieces.) Holland, " 'If You Know I Have a History,' " treats a section of *Almanac*. See also Van Dyke, "From Big Green Fly to the Stone Serpent," and St. Clair, "Death of Love/Love of Death." Now, with the publication of Barnett and Thorsen's *Collection of Critical Essays*, several dissertations, and more articles, there are more than forty scholarly publications that deal with *Almanac of the Dead*.

4. Birkerts, "Apocalypse Now," 39. He goes on to criticize the novel's "premise of revolutionary insurrection" as being "tethered to airy nothing" (41) in a withering review.

5. Silko, "Language and Literature from a Pueblo Indian Perspective," 83.

6. Coltelli, "Interview." In this interview Silko also describes the novel's structure as a "spiral," where "every story or single character is somehow connected with the other" (67).

7. See Silko, "Notes on *Almanac of the Dead*," in *Yellow Woman and a Beauty of the Spirit*, in which she discusses writing the novel and especially her notions of time as round, "like a tortilla" in which all times exist "side by side for all eternity" (137).

8. I have been asked on several occasions whether I believe this is a dystopian novel. I am uneasy about relegating *Almanac* solely to the realm of dystopia, although it certainly reflects on the systemic causes of social evil, as do dystopian novels. It is also realistic, and yet is the world as horrible as Silko's novel suggests? The one I inhabit mostly is not, but it bears a frightening resemblance at times. An important truth resides in Silko's vision of technology run amok and the move forward of the dispossessed to retake and heal the land, which, in fact, tilts this novel more in the direction of the utopian, depending on one's point of view. That is, for the dispossessed and their allies, this novel is actually more utopian than dystopian, a novel of daring dreams and radical hope. The text calls readers to take a careful look at our positionalities and with whom we align ourselves.

9. Coltelli, "Interview," 65.

10. Ward Churchill reports that Bernard Neitschmann surveyed armed conflicts occurring in 1988 alone and found that "of the 125 or so 'hot wars' he catalogued, fully eighty-five percent were being waged by specific indigenous peoples, or amalgamations of indigenous peoples against one or more nation-states . . . which claimed traditional native territories as their own" (Churchill, "North American Indigenist View," 151). Although, in Silko's world, the reclamation of land will take years, *Almanac* implicitly challenges readers to think now about the notion of solidarity and where one stands in relation to the world's oppressed people.

11. All quotations from Silko, *Almanac*, will be cited parenthetically in the text.

12. The Spanish word for spike or hook is *escarpia*.

13. Silko has mentioned in interviews how funny the novel is. It took me a second or even third reading to find the humor, so overwhelming were the representations of social decline, but at times the novel is, indeed, hilarious.

14. Careful readers will note that the eco-warriors also appear in the preceding paragraph describing "forces for good" that appear in the novel. This is one of the complexities of *Almanac*'s world (and ours as well): there are no clear heroes, although there are some who are clearly villains.

15. Krupat, *Voice in the Margin*, 55.

16. King, "New Epic for an Old World," 39.

17. Lock, "Displacing Suffering," 208.

18. Commenting on *Ceremony*, Lisa Orr, in "Theorizing the Earth," 149, points out that "technology becomes merely the stopgap that whites use to fill up the emptiness left after 'the lies devoured white hearts.' " Orr also develops the connection between *Ceremony* and *Almanac* around Silko's concepts of technological progress and nature.

19. See Fox and Swazey's *Spare Parts*, esp. 3–30, for a rich detailing of the effects of immunosuppressive drugs on transplant technology. Although neither cyclosporine nor FK 506 have become the miracle drugs they were first assumed to be, they and other immunosuppressives have made possible more organ transplants than ever before.

20. Ibid., 45.

21. Evans, "Organ Procurement Expenditures." Evans notes that in 1986, for example, 8,972 persons awaited kidney transplant; the number increased to 23,586 just seven years later in 1993. Numbers for liver transplants rose from 289 to 2,644; for hearts, the figure grew from 282 to 2,840. The total number of those awaiting kidney, liver, pancreas, heart, heart-lung, and lung transplants went from 9,632 in 1986 to 31,333 in 1993.

22. DuRivage, "Animal Farm."

23. Spital and Erin, "Conscription of Cadaveric Organs." The authors argue that consent is not ethically required for harvest of cadaveric organs and that, given the urgent need, a conscription system is ethically indicated.

24. Barnett and Kaserman, "Shortage of Organs for Transplantation," 120.

25. See, e.g., Horton and Horton, "Improving the Current System for Supplying Organs for Transplantation"; Prottas, "Encouraging Altruism"; Hansmann, "Economics and Ethics of Markets for Human Organs"; Maverodes, "Morality of Selling Human Organs"; Fluss, "Commerce in Human Organs"; Mark T. Nelson, "Morality of a Free Market"; Rosner et al., "Ethical and Social Issues in Organ Procurement"; Schlitt, "Paid Non-Related Living Organ Donation"; Shannon, "Kindness of Strangers."

26. Fox and Swazey, *Spare Parts*, 65. Jacobs's gambit led to the 1984 National Organ Transplantation Act that established networks for organ procurement and outlawed commercial markets in transplantable organs. Susan Hankin Denise also discusses the Jacobs case in "Regulating the Sale of Human Organs."

27. Seyfer, "eBay Halts Bidding for Kidney." What is particularly telling is that

the kidney was offered initially at $25,000 on August 26, and by September 2, when eBay pulled the ad, the price had risen to $5.7 million. Whether or not the offering was a prank, the interest was intense. The description read, "Fully functional kidney for sale. You can choose either kidney. Buyer pays all transplant and medical costs. Of course only one for sale, as I need the other one to live. Serious bids only." The auction was stopped, according to a company spokesperson, because "the seller broke eBay's rules outlawing the sale of body parts."

28. In addition, Serlo has funded a Swiss scientist to construct an "Alternative Earth module, loaded with the last of the earth's uncontaminated soil, water, and oxygen [to] be launched by immense rockets into high orbits around the earth where sunlight would sustain plants to supply oxygen as well as food" (Silko, *Almanac*, 542). These modules would be self-sufficient, closed systems where the wealthy would look down on earth until the upheaval and violence that "threatened those of superior lineage" finally ended (ibid., 543).

29. Patricia A. Marshall, "Organ Transplantation in Egypt."

30. Bauman, *Mortality, Immortality, and Other Life Strategies*, 131. My thanks to Nancy M. P. King for calling my attention to Bauman and the relevance of his thinking to this project.

31. Ibid., 155.

32. Fox and Swazey, *Spare Parts*, 40.

33. Also, in 1971 Titmuss had argued in *Gift Relation* against the commodification of human blood for both economic and philosophical reasons.

34. Fox and Swazey, *Spare Parts*, 67.

35. Patricia A. Marshall points out in "Organ Transplantation in Egypt," 21, that "the expansion of western scientific technology has been characterized as a new kind of imperialism."

36. There is, of course, a precedent for this in the United States. After abolition, the bodies of dead convicts (many of whom were former slaves) were sold to medical schools in Tennessee, for example. See Franklin, introduction.

37. Leah, for example is utterly convinced that technology will solve the problems of the extreme drought plaguing the Southwest (and thus add substantially to her wealth). Planning to build a dream city of Venetian canals and multimillion-dollar homes, "calculated with Arizona's financial collapse and Mexico's civil war in mind" (Silko, *Almanac*, 662), Leah can only do so by relying on technology to provide the water by drilling dangerously deep wells, a scheme vigorously opposed by local environmental groups. She insists, however, that "science will solve the water problem of the West. New technology. They'll *have* to" (ibid., 374).

38. Another novel that works similarly is Richard Powers's *Operation Wandering Soul*, in which a pediatric surgeon in a large public hospital in Los Angeles is confronted with the agonies of his patients' lives and diseases and begins to understand them in the broader context of the horrors of war and global poverty.

39.   Niemann, "New World Disorder," 1–4.

40.   Annas, "Questing for Grails," 328.

Chapter 8

1.   All quotations from Butler, *Parable of the Sower* and *Parable of the Talents*, will be cited parenthetically within the text.

2.   Zaki, "Future Tense," 37.

3.   Potts, " 'We Keep Playing the Same Record,' " 334.

4.   Mehaffy and Keating, "Radio Imagination," 47.

5.   Ibid., 74.

6.   Moylan, *Scraps of the Untainted Sky*, 196.

7.   Ibid., xi, xiii.

8.   Ibid., xv.

9.   In their interview with Octavia Butler, Mehaffy and Keating characterize *Sower* and *Talents* as exploring "physical and psychic forms of subjugation" ("Radio Imagination," 74).

10.   Turner, *Ritual Process*, 94.

11.   Ibid.

12.   Ibid., 96.

13.   Ibid., 97.

14.   Ibid., 113.

15.   Ibid., 131–32.

16.   Jehlen, "Gender," 271.

17.   World Health Organization, "Constitution."

18.   Mann et al., "Health and Human Rights," 8.

19.   Potts, " 'We Keep Playing the Same Record,' " 334.

20.   This is Lauren's interpretation. Butler, in an interview, states that hyperempathy syndrome is a "crippling delusion" of Lauren's and not based in any systemic reality, raising the issue of the mind/body connection of illness, one to which I think Butler gives much shorter shrift in the interview than she does in the novel, where Lauren's hyperempathy syndrome is much more complicated than simply standing as a "delusion." See ibid., 335.

21.   Butler tempers naive optimism with Larkin's continuing contempt for Earthseed. Indeed, the question of Earthseed's destiny residing in the stars exists in tension with Larkin's point of view: "The more I read about Earthseed, the more I despised it. So much needed to be done here on earth— so many diseases, so much hunger, so much poverty, such suffering, and here was a rich organization spending vast sums of money, time, and effort on nonsense. Just nonsense!" (Butler, *Talents*, 340–41). Butler only provides slight tension, however; Lauren's vision is sound, and the community thrives despite Larkin's contempt for it. Earthseed also seems to have done more than its share in creating something good out of the Pox and Christian America's repressive menu of so-called solutions.

22.   Dubey, "Folk and Urban Communities," 112; emphasis mine.

Coda

1. Sharf et al., " 'So Your Main Concern Is Getting This Pain under Control.' "
2. Mann, "Medicine and Public Health," 439–52.
3. Ibid., 451.
4. See, e.g, White, *Black Women's Health Book*; Roberts, "Reconstructing the Patient"; Warshaw, "Domestic Violence"; Sherwin, *No Longer Patient*; Waitzkin, *Politics of Medical Encounters*.

Bibliography

Abraham, Laurie Kaye. *Mama Might Be Better Off Dead: The Failure of Health Care in Urban America*. Chicago: University of Chicago Press, 1993.

Ad Hoc Committee to Defend Health Care. "For Our Patients, Not for Profits: A Call to Action." In *Health and Human Rights: A Reader*, edited by Jonathan M. Mann, Sofia Gruskin, Michael A. Grodin, and George J. Annas, 436–38. New York: Routledge, 1999.

Allen, Paula Gunn. "The Feminine Landscape of Leslie Marmon Silko's *Ceremony*." *Studies in American Indian Literature* 10.3 (1986): 121–33.

———. *The Sacred Hoop: Recovering the Feminine in American Indian Traditions*. Boston: Beacon Press, 1992.

Angelou, Maya. *I Know Why the Caged Bird Sings*. New York: Bantam, 1971.

Annas, George J. "Questing for Grails: Duplicity, Betrayal, and Self-Deception in Postmodern Medical Research." In *Health and Human Rights: A Reader*, edited by Jonathan M. Mann, Sofia Gruskin, Michael A. Grodin, and George J. Annas, 312–35. New York: Routledge, 1999.

Antell, Judith. "Momaday, Welch, and Silko: Expressing the Feminine Principle through Male Alienation." *American Indian Quarterly* 5.1 (1971): 7–12.

Anzaldúa, Gloria, *Borderlands/La Frontera: The New Mestiza*. San Francisco: Aunt Lute Books, 1987.

———, ed. *Making Face, Making Soul: Haciendo Caras: Creative and Critical Perspectives by Feminists of Color*. San Francisco: Aunt Lute Books, 1990.

Atwood, Margaret. *Bodily Harm*. New York: Simon and Schuster, 1982.

———. *The Handmaid's Tale*. Boston: Houghton Mifflin, 1986.

Awkward, Michael. "Authorial Dreams of Wholeness: (Dis)Unity, (Literary) Parentage, and *The Women of Brewster Place*." In *Gloria Naylor: Critical Perspectives Past and Present*, edited by Henry Louis Gates Jr. and K. A. Appiah, 37–70. New York: Amistad Press, 1993.

Bakhtin, M. M. "Epic and Novel." In *The Dialogic Novel: Essays by M. M. Bakhtin*, edited by Michael Holquist, 3–40. Austin: University of Texas Press, 1981.

Bambara, Toni Cade. *The Salt Eaters*. New York: Vintage, 1981.

———. "Salvation Is the Issue." In *Black Women Writers, 1950–1980: A Critical Evaluation*, edited by Mari Evans, 41–47. Garden City, N.Y.: Anchor, 1984.

Barnett, A. H., and D. L. Kaserman. "The Shortage of Organs for Transplantation: Exploring the Alternatives." *Issues in Law and Medicine* 19.2 (1993): 117–37.

Barnett, Louise K., and James L. Thorsen, eds. *Leslie Marmon Silko: A*

Collection of Critical Essays. Albuquerque: University of New Mexico Press, 1999.

Bauman, Zygmunt. *Mortality, Immortality, and Other Life Strategies*. Stanford: Stanford University Press, 1992.

Bell, Marilynne, and Janet Mosher. "(Re)fashioning Medicine's Response to Wife Abuse." In *The Politics of Women's Health: Exploring Agency and Autonomy*, edited by Susan Sherwin and the Feminist Health Care Ethics Research Network, 205–33. Philadelphia: Temple University Press, 1998.

Bellah, Robert, Richard Madsen, William M. Sullivan, Ann Swidler, Steven M. Tipton. *Habits of the Heart: Individualism and Commitment in American Life*. New York: Harper, 1985.

Bennett, Paula. "The Mother's Part: Incest and Deprivation in Woolf and Morrison." In *Narrating Mothers: Theorizing Maternal Subjectivities*, edited by Brenda O. Daly and Maureen T. Reddy, 125–38. Knoxville: University of Tennessee Press, 1991.

Berger, James. "Ghosts of Liberalism: Morrison's *Beloved* and the Moynihan Report." *PMLA* 3.3 (May 1996): 408–20.

Bevis, William. "Native American Novels: Homing In." In *Recovering the Word: Essays on Native American Literature*, edited by Brian Swann and Arnold Krupat, 580–620. Berkeley: University of California Press, 1987.

Bird, Gloria. "Towards a Decolonization of the Mind and Text 1: Leslie Marmon Silko's *Ceremony*." *Wicazo sa Review* 9.2 (1993): 1–8.

Birkerts, Sven. "Apocalypse Now." *New Republic*, no. 205 (November 1991): 39–41.

Bonner, Marita. *Frye Street and Environs*. Boston: Beacon Press, 1987.

Bordo, Susan. *Unbearable Weight: Feminism, Western Culture, and the Body*. Berkeley: University of California Press, 1993.

Brodber, Erna. *Jane and Louisa Will Soon Come Home*. London: New Beacon Books, 1980.

Brody, Howard. *The Healer's Power*. New Haven: Yale University Press, 1992.

——. *Stories of Sickness*. New Haven: Yale University Press, 1987.

——. "Who Gets to Tell the Story? Narrative In Postmodern Bioethics." In *Stories and Their Limits: Narrative Approaches to Bioethics*, edited by Hilde Lindemann Nelson, 18–30. New York: Routledge, 1997.

Brooks, Gwendolyn. "The Anniad." In *Annie Allen*, 19–29. New York: Harper and Brothers, 1949. Reprinted in Brooks, *Blacks*, 99–109. Chicago: David Press, 1994.

——. "Gay Chaps at the Bar." In *A Street in Bronzeville*, 46–57. New York: Harper and Brothers, 1945. Reprinted in Brooks, *Blacks*, 64–75. Chicago: David Press, 1994.

——. *Blacks*. Chicago: David Press, 1994.

Brown, Karen McCarthy. "Afro-Caribbean Spirituality: A Haitian Case Study." In *Healing and Restoring: Health and Medicine in the World's Religious Traditions*, edited by Lawrence E. Sullivan, 255–85. New York: Macmillan, 1989.

Brumberg, Joan Jacobs. *Fasting Girls: The Emergence of Anorexia Nervosa as a Modern Disease*. Cambridge: Harvard University Press, 1988.

Busia, Abena P. A. "What Is Your Nation?: Reconnecting Africa and Her Diaspora through Paule Marshall's *Praisesong for the Widow.*" In *Changing Our Own Words: Essays on Criticism, Theory, and Writing by Black Women,* edited by Cheryl A. Wall, 196–211. New Brunswick, N.J.: Rutgers University Press, 1989.

Butler, Octavia. *Parable of the Sower.* New York: Four Walls, Eight Windows, 1993.

———. *Parable of the Talents.* New York: Seven Stories Press, 1998.

Butler-Evans, Eliott, *Race, Gender, and Desire: Narrative Strategies in the Fiction of Toni Cade Bambara, Toni Morrison, and Alice Walker.* Philadelphia: Temple University Press, 1989.

Campbell, Bebe Moore. *Your Blues Ain't Like Mine: A Novel.* New York: Ballantine/Random House, 1993.

Cane, Patricia. ⟨www.capacitar.org⟩.

Carbonell, Ana Maria. "From Llorona to Gritona: Coatlicue in Feminist Tales by Viramontes and Cisneros." *MELUS* 21.2 (1999): 53–73.

Cassell, Eric. "The Nature of Suffering and the Goals of Medicine." *New England Journal of Medicine,* March 18, 1982, 639–45.

Castillo, Ana. *Massacre of the Dreamers: Essays on Xicanisma.* New York: Penguin/Plume, 1995.

———. *So Far from God.* New York: Penguin/Plume, 1994.

Castillo, Susan Pérez. "Postmodernism, Native American Literature, and the Real: The Silko-Erdrich Controversy." *Massachusetts Review,* Summer 1991, 285–94.

Chambers, Tod. "From the Ethicist's Point of View: The Literary Nature of Medical Ethics Cases." *Hastings Center Report* 26 (1996): 25–32.

Chao, Patricia. *Monkey King.* New York: HarperCollins, 1997.

Charon, Rita. "Narrative Contributions to Medical Ethics: Recognition, Formulation, Interpretation, and Validation in the Practice of the Ethicist." In *A Matter of Principles? Ferment in U.S. Bioethics,* edited by E. R. DuBose, R. P. Hamel, and L. J. O'Connell. Valley Forge, Pa.: Trinity Press, 1994.

Charon, Rita, Howard Brody, Mary Williams Clark, Dwight Davis, Richard Martinez, Robert M. Nelson. "Literature and Ethical Medicine: Five Cases from Common Practice." *Journal of Medicine and Philosophy* 21.3 (June 1996): 243–65.

Chernin, Kim. *The Hungry Self: Women, Eating, and Identity.* New York: Times Books, 1985.

———. *The Obsession: Reflections on the Tyranny of Slenderness.* New York: Harper and Row, 1981.

Christian, Barbara. *Black Feminist Criticism: Perspectives on Black Women Writers.* New York: Pergamon Press, 1985.

———. "The Contemporary Fables of Toni Morrison." In *Toni Morrison: Critical Perspectives Past and Present,* edited by Henry Louis Gates Jr. and K. A. Appiah, 59–99. New York: Amistad Press, 1993.

———. "Gloria Naylor's Geography: Community, Class, and Patriarchy in *The Women of Brewster Place* and *Linden Hills.*" In *Reading Black, Reading Feminist: A Critical Anthology,* edited by Henry Louis Gates Jr., 348–73. New York: Meridian, 1990.

Churchill, Ward, "A North American Indigenist View." In *First World, Ha Ha Ha!,* edited by Elaine Katzenberger, 141–55. San Francisco: City Lights Press, 1995.

Cisneros, Sandra. *Woman Hollering Creek and Other Stories.* New York: Vintage, 1991, 1992.

Clarke, Cheryl. "An Identity of One's Own." *Harvard Gay and Lesbian Review* 3 (Fall 1996): 37–38.

Clouser, K. Danner. "Philosophy, Literature, and Ethics: Let the Engagement Begin." *Journal of Medicine and Philosophy* 21.3 (June 1996): 321–40.

Cocteau, Jean. *Opium: The Diary of a Cure.* London: Peter Owen, 1957.

Cofer, Judith Ortiz. *The Line of the Sun.* Athens: University of Georgia Press, 1989.

Coltelli, Laura, "*Almanac of the Dead:* An Interview with Leslie Marmon Silko." *Native American Literature Forum* 4–5 (1992–93): 65–79.

Crow Dog, Mary, and Richard Erdoes. *Lakota Woman.* New York: Harper/Perennial, 1990.

Danticat, Edwidge. *Breath, Eyes, Memory.* New York: Vintage, 1995.

Das, Veena. "Language and Body: Transactions in the Construction of Pain." *Daedalus* 125.1 (Winter 1996): 67–93.

Davis, Angela Y. "Sick and Tired of Being Sick and Tired." In *The Black Women's Health Book: Speaking for Ourselves,* edited by Evelyn C. White, 18–26. Seattle: Seal Press, 1990.

Denise, Susan Hankin. "Regulating the Sale of Human Organs." *Virginia Law Review* 71 (1985): 1015–38.

Divakaruni, Chitra Bannerjee. *The Mistress of Spices.* New York: Anchor, 1997.

Doyle, Jacqueline, "Haunting the Borderlands: La Llorona in Sandra Cisneros's 'Woman Hollering Creek.'" *Frontiers: A Journal of Women's Studies* 16.1 (1996): 53–70.

Dubey, Madhu. "Folk and Urban Communities in African-American Women's Fiction: Octavia Butler's *Parable of the Sower.*" *Studies in American Fiction* 27.1 (Spring 1999): 103–28.

duRivage, J. "Animal Farm: The Ethics and Public Policy of Xenotransplantation." *Princeton Journal of Bioethics* 3.1 (Spring 2000): 8–19.

Ellison, Ralph. *Invisible Man.* 1952. New York: Vintage, 1990.

———. "Out of the Hospital and under the Bar." In *Soon, One Morning: New Writing by American Negroes, 1940–1962,* edited by Herbert Hill, 242–90. New York: Knopf, 1963.

Elshtain, Jean Bethke. *Women and War.* New York: Basic Books, 1987.

Engel, George. "The Biopsychosocial Model and the Education of Health Professionals." *Annals of the New York Academy of Sciences,* June 21, 1978, 169–81.

———. "The Need for a New Medical Model: A Challenge for Biomedicine." *Science,* April 8, 1977, 129–36.

Erdrich, Louise. *The Beet Queen.* New York: Henry Holt, 1986.

———. *The Bingo Palace.* New York: Harper/Perennial, 1995.

———. *Love Medicine.* New York: HarperCollins, 1984.

——. *Tracks*. New York: Harper/Perennial, 1989.

Evans, Roger W. "Organ Procurement Expenditures and the Role of Financial Incentives." *Journal of the American Medical Association* 269.24 (1993): 3113–18.

Fabri, Mary R. "A Clinical Perspective of the Role of Gender in the Torture Experience." Unpublished manuscript. March 1999.

Fadiman, Anne. *The Spirit Catches You and You Fall Down: A Hmong Child, Her American Doctors, and the Collision of Two Cultures*. New York: Farrar, Strauss and Giroux/Noonday: 1997.

Fanon, Frantz. *The Wretched of the Earth*. New York: Grove Press, 1968.

Farmer, Paul. "Listening for Prophetic Voices in Medicine." *America*, July 5–7, 1997, 8–13.

——. "On Suffering and Structural Violence: A View from Below." *Daedalus* 125.1 (Winter 1996): 261–83.

Ferraro, Kathleen J. "The Dance of Dependency: A Genealogy of Domestic Violence Discourse." *Hypatia* 11.4 (Fall 1996): 76–91.

Flores, Toni. "Claiming and Making: Ethnicity, Gender, and the Common Sense in Leslie Marmon Silko's *Ceremony* and Zora Neale Hurston's *Their Eyes Were Watching God*." *Frontiers: A Journal of Women's Studies* 10.3 (1989): 52–58.

Fluss, Sev S. "Commerce in Human Organs: The International Response." *World Health Forum* 12.3 (1991): 307–10.

Foucault, Michel. "Two Lectures." In *Power/Knowledge: Selected Interviews and Other Writings, 1972–1977*, edited by Colin Gordon, 78–108. New York: Pantheon, 1980.

Fox, Renee C., and Judith P. Swazey. *Spare Parts: Organ Replacement in American Society*. New York: Oxford University Press, 1992.

Fraden, Rena. *Imagining Medea: Rhodessa Jones and Theater for Incarcerated Women*. Chapel Hill: University of North Carolina Press, 2001.

Frank, Arthur. "Enacting Illness Stories: When, What, and Why." In *Stories and Their Limits: Narrative Approaches to Bioethics*, edited by Hilde Lindemann Nelson, 31–49. New York: Routledge, 1997.

——. *The Wounded Storyteller: Body, Illness, and Ethics*. Chicago: University of Chicago Press, 1995.

Franklin, H. Bruce, ed. Introduction to *Prison Writing in Twentieth Century America*, 1–18. New York: Penguin, 1998.

Freire, Paulo. *Pedagogy of the Oppressed*. New York: Herder and Herder, 1970.

Furst, Lilian, and Peter W. Graham, eds. *Disorderly Eaters: Texts in Self-Empowerment*. University Park: Pennsylvania State University Press, 1992.

Garcia, Reyes. "Senses of Place in *Ceremony*." *MELUS* 10.4 (1983): 37–48.

Gurganus, Allan. *The Oldest Living Confederate Widow Tells All*. New York: Knopf/Random House, 1989.

Handley, William R. "The House a Ghost Built: Nommo, Allegory, and the Ethics of Reading in Toni Morrison's *Beloved*." *Contemporary Literature* 36.4 (1995): 676–701.

Hansmann, H. "The Economics and Ethics of Markets for Human Organs." *Journal of Health Politics, Policy, and Law* 14.1 (1989): 57–85.

Harjo, Joy. "The World Is Round: Some Notes on Leslie Silko's *Almanac of the Dead*." *Blue Mesa Review* 4 (Spring 1992): 207–12.

Harris, Trudier. "From Exile to Asylum: Religion and Community in the Writings of Contemporary Black Women." In *Women's Writing in Exile*, edited by Mary Lynn Broe and Angela Ingram, 151–69. Chapel Hill: University of North Carolina Press, 1989.

Hawkins, Anne Hunsaker. "Literature, Philosophy, and Medical Ethics: Let the Dialogue Go On." *Journal of Medicine and Philosophy* 21.3 (June 1996): 341–54.

Hearn, Melissa. "Review: *Almanac of the Dead*." *Prairie Schooner* 67.2 (Summer 1993): 149–51.

Heberle, Renee. "Deconstructive Strategies and the Movement against Sexual Violence." *Hypatia* 11.4 (Fall 1996): 63–75.

Henderson, Gail E., Nancy M. P. King, Ronald P. Strauss, Sue E. Estroff, and Larry R. Churchill, eds. *The Social Medicine Reader*. Durham, N.C.: Duke University Press, 1997.

Henderson, Mae G. "Toni Morrison's *Beloved*: Re-Membering the Body as Historical Text." In *Comparative American Identities: Race, Sex, and Nationality in the Modern Text*, ed. Hortense J. Spillers, 62–86. New York: Routledge, 1991.

Herman, Judith. *Trauma and Recovery: The Aftermath of Violence—from Domestic Abuse to Political Terror*. New York: Basic Books, 1992, 1997.

Hilfiker, David. *Healing the Wounds: A Physician Looks at His Work*. New York: Viking/Penguin, 1987.

Hoagland, Sarah. *Lesbian Ethics: Toward New Value*. Palo Alto, Calif.: Institute of Lesbian Studies, 1988.

Hogeland, C., and Rosen, K. A. "A Needs Assessment of Undocumented Women." March 1990. Study available from the Northern California Coalition for Immigrant Rights, 995 Market Street, 11th Floor, San Francisco, CA 94103.

Holland, Sharon P. " 'If You Know I Have a History, You Will Respect Me': A Perspective on Afro-Native American Literature." *Callaloo: A Journal of African American and African Arts and Letters* 17.1 (Winter 1994): 334–50.

Hollar, M. C. "The Impact of Racism on the Delivery of Health Care and Mental Health Services." *Psychiatric Quarterly* 72.4 (Winter 2001): 337–45.

Holloway, Karla F. C. *Moorings and Metaphors: Figures of Culture and Gender in Black Women's Literature*. New Brunswick, N.J.: Rutgers University Press, 1992.

hooks, bell. *Black Looks: Race and Representation*. Boston: South End Press, 1992.

——. "Living to Love." In *The Black Women's Health Book: Speaking for Ourselves*, edited by Evelyn C. White, 332–41. Seattle: Seal Press, 1990.

——. "Narratives of Struggle." In *Critical Fictions: The Politics of Imaginative Writing*, edited by Philomena Mariani, 53–61. Seattle: Bay Press, 1991.

Horton, Raymond L., and Patricia J. Horton. "Improving the Current System for Supplying Organs for Transplantation." *Journal of Health Politics, Policy, and Law* 18.1 (1993): 175–87.

Hulme, Keri. *The Bone People*. Baton Rouge: Louisiana State University Press, 1985.

Hunter, Kathryn Montgomery. "Making a Case." Introduction by D. Heywood Broun. *Literature and Medicine* 7 (1988): 64–79.

———. "Narrative." In *Encyclopedia of Bioethics*, edited by Warren T. Reich, 1789–93. New York: Simon and Schuster, Macmillan, 1993.

Hurston, Zora Neale. *Mules and Men*. 1935. Bloomington: Indiana University Press, 1978.

———. *Tell My Horse*. 1937. Berkeley, Calif: Turtle Island, 1981.

———. *Their Eyes Were Watching God*. 1938. Urbana: University of Illinois Press, 1978.

Hurtado, Aída. "Strategic Suspensions: Feminists of Color Theorize the Production of Knowledge." In *Knowledge, Difference, and Power: Essays Inspired by Women's Ways of Knowing*, edited by Nancy Goldberger, Jill Tarule, Blythe Clinchy, and Mary Belenky, 372–92. New York: Basic Books, 1996.

Jehlen, Myra. "Gender." In *Critical Terms for Literary Study*, edited by Frank Lentricchia and Thomas McLaughlin, 263–73. Chicago: University of Chicago Press, 1990.

Jones, Anne Hudson. "Darren's Case: Narrative Ethics in Perri Klass's *Other Women's Children*." *Journal of Medicine and Philosophy* 21.3 (June 1996): 267–86.

Jones, Gayl. *Corregidora*. 1975. Boston: Beacon Press, 1986.

———. *Eva's Man*. 1976. Boston: Beacon Press, 1987.

———. *The Healing*. Boston: Beacon Press, 1998.

Kavanaugh, Kieran, and Otillo Rodriguez. *The Collected Works of St. Teresa of Avila*. Vol. 1. Washington, D.C.: Institute of Carmelite Studies, 1976.

Kesey, Ken. *One Flew over the Cuckoo's Nest*. New York: Viking, 1973.

King, Katherine Callen. "New Epic for an Old World: Leslie Marmon Silko's *Almanac of the Dead*." *Native American Literature Forum* 4–5 (1992–93): 31–42.

Kleinman, Arthur. *The Illness Narratives: Suffering, Healing, and the Human Condition*. New York: Basic Books, 1988.

———. "Pain and Resistance: The Delegitimation and Relegitimation of Local Worlds." In *Pain as Human Experience: An Anthropological Perspective*, edited by Mary-Jo Delvecchio Good, Paul E. Brodwin, Byron J. Good, and Arthur Kleinman, 169–97. Berkeley: University of California Press, 1992.

———. *Writing at the Margin: Discourse between Anthropology and Medicine*. Berkeley: University of California Press, 1995.

Kleinman, Arthur, and Joan Kleinman. "The Appeal of Experience: The Dismay of Images: Cultural Appropriations of Suffering in Our Times." *Daedalus* 125.1 (Winter 1996): 1–24.

Koolish, Lynda. "Fictive Strategies and Cinematic Representations in Toni Morrison's *Beloved*: Postcolonial Theory/Postcolonial Text." *African American Review* 29.3 (1995): 421–38.

Krupat, Arnold. *The Voice in the Margin: Native American Literature and the Canon.* Los Angeles: University of California Press, 1989.

Laub, Dori. "Bearing Witness, or the Vicissitudes of Listening." In *Testimony: Crises of Witnessing in Literature, Psychoanalysis, and History*, edited by Shoshana Felman and Dori Laub, 57–74. New York: Routledge, 1992.

LeClair, Thomas. "The Language Must Not Sweat: A Conversation with Toni Morrison." *New Republic*, no. 21 (March 1981): 25–29.

Lelwica, Michelle Mary. *Starving for Salvation: The Spiritual Dimensions of Eating Problems among American Girls.* New York: Oxford University Press, 1999.

Lock, Margaret. "Displacing Suffering: The Reconstruction of Death in North America and Japan." *Daedalus* 125.1 (Winter 1996): 207–44.

Mann, Jonathan M. "Medicine and Public Health, Ethics, and Human Rights." In *Health and Human Rights: A Reader*, edited by Jonathan M. Mann, Sofia Gruskin, Michael A. Grodin, and George J. Annas, 439–52. New York: Routledge, 1999.

Mann, Jonathan M., Lawrence Gostin, Sofia Gruskin, Troyen Brennan, Zita Lazzarini, and Harvey Fineberg. "Health and Human Rights." In *Health and Human Rights: A Reader*, edited by Jonathan M. Mann, Sofia Gruskin, Michael A. Grodin, and George J. Annas, 7–20. New York: Routledge, 1999.

Marshall, Patricia A. "Organ Transplantation in Egypt: The Concept of Ownership and the Problem of Consent." Unpublished manuscript. June 28, 1994.

Marshall, Paule. *Praisesong for the Widow.* New York: Obelisk/Dutton, 1983.

Maverodes, George. "The Morality of Selling Human Organs." *Progressive Clinical and Biological Research* 38 (1989): 133–39.

McClusky, John, Jr. "And Called Every Generation Blessed: Theme, Setting, and Ritual in the Works of Paule Marshall." In *Black Women Writers, 1950–1980: A Critical Evaluation*, edited by Mari Evans, 316–34. Garden City, N.Y.: Anchor, 1984.

McLeer, S. V., and R. Anwar. "A Study of Women Presenting in an Emergency Department." *American Journal of Public Health* 79 (1989): 65–67.

Mehaffy, Marilyn, and AnaLouise Keating. " 'Radio Imagination': Octavia Butler on the Poetics of Narrative Embodiment." *MELUS* 26.1 (2001): 45–76.

Meisenhelder, Susan. " 'The Whole Picture' in Gloria Naylor's *Mama Day*." *African American Review* 27.3 (1993): 405–19.

Melville, Herman, *White-Jacket; or, The World in a Man-of-War.* 1850. Edited by Hayford Harrison, Hershel Parker, and G. Thomas Tanselle. Evanston, Ill.: Northwestern University Press, 2000.

Melzack, Ronald, and Patrick D. Wall. *The Challenge of Pain.* New York: Basic Books, 1973.

Montello, Martha. "Narrative Competence." In *Stories and Their Limits: Narrative Approaches to Bioethics*, edited by Hilde Lindemann Nelson, 185–97. New York: Routledge, 1997.

Moran, Patricia, and Tamar Heller. *Scenes of the Apple: Food and the Female*

Body in Nineteenth and Twentieth Century Women's Writing. Albany: SUNY Press, forthcoming.

Morris, David. *The Culture of Pain.* Berkeley: University of California Press, 1991.

Morrison, R. Sean, Sylvan Wallenstein, Dana K. Natale, Richard S. Senzel, and Lo-Li Huang. " 'We Don't Carry That': Failure of Pharmacies in Predominantly Nonwhite Neighborhoods to Stock Opioid Analgesics." *New England Journal of Medicine,* April 6, 2000, 1023–26.

Morrison, Toni. *Beloved.* New York: Knopf, 1987.

———. *The Bluest Eye.* New York: Holt, Rhinehart, and Winston, 1970.

Moylan, Tom. *Scraps of the Untainted Sky: Science Fiction, Utopia, Dystopia.* Boulder, Colo.: Westview, 2000.

Mullen, Harryette. "A Silence between Us Like Language: The Untranslatability of Experience in Sandra Cisneros's 'Woman Hollering Creek.' " *MELUS* 21.5 (1996): 3–20.

Naylor, Gloria. *Bailey's Café.* Orlando, Fla.: Harcourt, Brace, Jovanovich, 1992.

———. *Mama Day.* New York: Vintage, 1989.

———. *The Women of Brewster Place.* New York: Penguin, 1983.

Nelson, Hilde Lindemann, ed. *Stories and Their Limits: Narrative Approaches to Bioethics.* New York: Routledge, 1997.

Nelson, Mark T. "The Morality of a Free Market for Transplant Organs." *Public Affairs Quarterly* 5 (1991): 63–79.

Nelson, Robert M. "Place and Vision: The Function of Landscape in *Ceremony.*" *Journal of the Southwest* 3 (1988): 281–316.

Ng, Bernardo, J. E. Dimsdale, G. P. Shragg, and R. Deutsch. "Ethnic Differences in Analgesic Consumption for Postoperative Pain." *Psychosomatic Medicine* 58.2 (March–April 1996): 125–29.

Niemann, Linda. "New World Disorder." *Women's Review of Books* 9.6 (March 1992): 1–4.

Orbach, Susie. *Fat Is a Feminist Issue: The Anti-Diet Guide to Permanent Weight Loss.* New York: Berkeley Books, 1978.

———. *Hunger Strike: The Anorectic's Struggle as a Metaphor for Our Age.* London: Faber, 1986.

Orr, Lisa, "Theorizing the Earth: Feminist Approaches to Nature and Leslie Marmon Silko's *Ceremony.*" *American Indian Culture and Research Journal* 18.2 (1994): 145–57.

Palmer, G. E. H., Philip Sherrard, and Kallistos Ware. *The Philokalia: The Complete Text Compiled by St. Nikodimos of the Holy Mountain and St. Makarios of Corinth.* Vol. 1. 1979. Boston: Faber and Faber, 1986.

Patchett, Ann. *The Magician's Assistant.* New York: Harcourt, Brace, 1997.

Pemberton, Gayle. "A Hunger for Language." *Women's Review of Books* 14.2 (November 1996): 1, 3.

Pernick, Martin S. *A Calculus of Suffering: Pain, Professionalism, and Anesthesia in Nineteenth Century America.* New York: Columbia University Press, 1985.

Perrone, Bobbette, H. Henrietta Stockel, and Victoria Krueger. *Medicine Women, Curanderas, and Women Doctors.* Norman: University of Oklahoma Press, 1989.

Peterson, Nancy J. "History, Postmodernism, and Louise Erdrich's *Tracks*." *PMLA* 109.5 (October 1994): 982–94.

Potts, Stephen W. " 'We Keep Playing the Same Record': A Conversation with Octavia E. Butler." *Science Fiction Studies* 23 (November 1996): 331–38.

Powers, Richard. *Operation Wandering Soul: A Novel.* New York: Morrow, 1993.

Prottas, J. M. "Encouraging Altruism: Public Attitudes and the Marketing of Organ Donation." *Milbank Memorial Fund Quarterly* 61.2 (1983): 278–306.

Rainwater, Catherine. "The Semiotics of Dwelling in Leslie Marmon Silko's *Ceremony*." *American Journal of Semiotics* 9.2–3 (1992): 219–40.

Rich, Adrienne. "If Not with Others, How?" In *Blood, Bread, and Poetry: Selected Prose, 1979–1985.* London: Virago, 1987.

Richie, Beth E. *Compelled to Crime: The Gender Entrapment of Battered Black Women.* New York: Routledge, 1996.

Ridley, C. R., D. W. Chih, and R. J. Olivera. "Training in Cultural Schemas: An Antidote to Unintentional Racism in Clinical Practice." *American Journal of Orthopsychiatry* 70.1 (January 2000): 65–72.

Riley, Patricia. "The Mixed Blood Writer as Interpreter and Mythmaker." In *Understanding Others: Cultural and Cross-Cultural Studies and the Teaching of Literature,* edited by Joseph Trimmer and Tilly Warnock, 230–42. Urbana, Ill.: National Council of Teachers of English, 1992.

Roberts, Dorothy. *Killing the Black Body: Race, Reproduction, and the Meaning of Liberty.* New York: Vintage, 1997.

——. "Reconstructing the Patient: Starting with Women of Color." In *Feminism and Bioethics: Beyond Reproduction,* edited by Susan M. Wolf, 116–43. New York: Oxford University Press, 1996.

Rollock, David, and Edmund W. Gordon. "Racism and Mental Health into the Twenty-first Century: Perspectives and Parameters." *American Journal of Orthopsychiatry* 70.1 (January 2000): 5–13.

Rosner, Fred, J. B. Henry, J. R. Wolpaw, P. P. Sordillo, P. H. Sechzer, P. Rogatz, H. M. Risemberg, F. V. Ona, P. J. Numann, and R. E. Lowenstein. "Ethical and Social Issues in Organ Procurement for Transplantation." *New York State Journal of Medicine* 93.1 (1993): 30–34.

Ruppert, James. "Dialogism and Mediation in Leslie Silko's *Ceremony*." *Explicator* 51.2 (Winter 1993): 129–34.

Russo, Ann. *Taking Back Our Lives: A Call to Action for the Feminist Movement.* New York: Routledge, 2001.

St. Andrews, B. A. "Healing the Witchery: Medicine in Silko's *Ceremony*." *Arizona Quarterly* 44.1 (1988): 86–94.

St. Clair, Janet. "Death of Love/Love of Death: Leslie Marmon Silko's *Almanac of the Dead*." *MELUS* 21.2 (1996): 141–58.

Sapphire, *Push.* New York: Vintage, 1997.

Sayles, John. Interview. http://www.spe.sonypictures.com/classics/menwithguns/production.html.

Scarberry, Susan J. "Memory as Medicine: The Power of Recollection in *Ceremony*." *American Indian Quarterly* 5.1 (1971): 19–26.

Scarry, Elaine. *The Body in Pain: The Making and Unmaking of a World.* New York: Oxford University Press, 1985.

Schapiro, Barbara. "The Bonds of Love and the Boundaries of Self in Toni Morrison's *Beloved.*" *Contemporary Literature* 32.2 (Summer 1991): 194–210.

Scheper-Hughes, Nancy. *Death without Weeping: The Violence of Everyday Life in Brazil.* Berkeley: University of California Press, 1992.

Schlitt, H. J. "Paid Non-Related Living Organ Donation: Horn of Plenty or Pandora's Box?" *Lancet,* March 16, 2002, 906–7.

Schweninger, Lee. "Writing Nature: Silko and Native Americans as Nature Writers." *MELUS* 18.2 (1993): 47–60.

Schwindt, R., and A. R. Vining. "Proposal for a Future Delivery Market for Transplant Organs." *Journal of Health Politics, Policy, and Law* 11.3 (1986): 483–500.

Scott, James C. *Domination and the Arts of Resistance: Hidden Transcripts.* New Haven: Yale University Press, 1990.

Seyfer, Jessie. "eBay Halts Bidding for Kidney." *Chicago Sun-Times,* September 3, 1999.

Shange, Ntozake. *for colored girls who have considered suicide / when the rainbow is enuf.* 1970. New York: Bantam, 1980.

Shannon, Thomas A. "The Kindness of Strangers: Organ Transplantation in a Capitalist Age." *Kennedy Institute of Ethics Journal* 11.3 (2001): 285–303.

Sharf, Barbara, Ann Folwell Stanford, Kathryn Montgomery, and John Kahler. "'So Your Main Concern Is Getting This Pain under Control': A Clinical Case as Text and Performance." Unpublished manuscript. August 1998.

Sherwin, Susan. *No Longer Patient: Feminist Ethics and Health Care.* Philadelphia: Temple University Press, 1992.

Silko, Leslie Marmon. *Almanac of the Dead: A Novel.* New York: Penguin, 1991.

———. *Ceremony.* New York: Viking/Penguin, 1977, 1986.

———. "Language and Literature from a Pueblo Indian Perspective." In *Critical Fictions: The Politics of Imaginative Writing,* edited by Philomena Mariani, 83–93. Seattle: Bay Press, 1991.

———. *Yellow Woman and a Beauty of the Spirit: Essays on Native American Life Today.* New York: Simon and Schuster, 1996.

Simon, Roger, and Jeffrey Manier. "Ravenswood Hospital Threatened by Clinton." *Chicago Tribune,* May 30, 1998.

Slowik, Mary. "Henry James, Meet Spider Woman: A Study of Narrative Form in Leslie Silko's *Ceremony.*" *Dakota Quarterly* 57.2 (1989): 104–29.

Snow, Loudell F. *Walkin' over Medicine.* Boulder, Colo.: Westview, 1993.

Spital, A., and C. A. Erin. "Conscription of Cadaveric Organs for Transplantation: Let's at Least Talk about It." *American Journal of Kidney Diseases* 39.3 (March 2002): 611–15.

Spurr, Stephen, "The Proposed Market for Human Organs." *American Journal of Kidney Diseases* 39.3 (March 2002): 189–202.

Stanford, Ann Folwell. "From the Mouth of Her Wound: Pain, Sexuality, and Resistance in Jean Stafford's 'The Interior Castle.'" *Women's Studies* 24 (1995): 585–97.

——. " 'Human Debris': Border Politics, Body Parts, and the Reclamation of the Americas in Leslie Marmon Silko's *Almanac of the Dead.*" *Literature and Medicine* 16.1 (Spring 1997): 23–42.

——. "Mechanisms of Disease: Health, Illness, and the Limits of Medicine in Three African-American Women's Novels." *NWSA Journal* 6.1 (1994): 28–47.

——. "Women's Advocacy and Healing in El Salvador." *Diálogo* 6 (Winter/Spring 2002): 49–50.

Storhoff, Gary. " 'The Only Voice Is Your Own': Gloria Naylor's Revision of 'The Tempest.' " *African American Review* 29.1 (1995): 35–45.

Stoudt, Debra L. "Medieval German Women and the Power of Healing." In *Women Healers and Physicians: Climbing a Long Hill,* edited by Lilian R. Furst, 13–42. Lexington: University Press of Kentucky, 1997.

Swan, Edith. "Feminine Perspectives at Laguna Pueblo: Silko's *Ceremony.*" *Tulsa Studies in Women's Literature* 11.2 (1992): 309–28.

Swartz, Sally. "Colonizing the Insane: Causes of Insanity in the Cape, 1891–1920." *History of the Human Sciences* 8.4 (1995): 39–57.

Tanner, Lindsey. "Teen Dies Near Hospital after Workers Refused to Help." Associated Press. May 19, 1998.

Taussig, Michael T. "Reification and the Consciousness of the Patient." *Social Science and Medicine* 14B (1980): 3–13.

Thomas, Maria. *Antonia Saw the Oryx First.* New York: Soho, 1987.

Thompson, Becky W. *A Hunger So Wide and So Deep: A Multiracial View of Women's Eating Problems.* Minneapolis: University of Minnesota Press, 1994.

Thompson, Robert Farris. *Flash of the Spirit: African and Afro-American Art and Philosophy.* New York: Random House, 1983.

Titmuss, Richard M. *The Gift Relation: From Human Body to Social Policy.* New York: Pantheon, 1971.

Titus, Mary. " 'This Poisonous System': Social Ills, Bodily Ills, and *Incidents in the Life of a Slave Girl.*" In *Harriet Jacobs and "Incidents in the Life of a Slave Girl": New Critical Essays,* edited by Deborah M. Garfield and Rafia Zafar, 199–215. New York: Cambridge University Press, 1996.

Tjaden, Patricia, and Nancy Thoennes. "Prevalence, Incidence, and Consequences of Violence against Women: Findings from the National Violence against Women Survey." NCJ 183781. November 2000. http://www.ncjrs.org/.

Todd, K. H., C. Deaton, A. P. D'Adamo, and L. Goe. "Ethnicity and Analgesic Practice." *Annals of Emergency Medicine,* January 2000, 11–16.

Traylor, Eleanor. "Music as Theme: The Jazz Mode in the Works of Toni Cade Bambara." In *Black Women Writers, 1950–1980: A Critical Evaluation,* edited by Mari Evans, 58–70. Garden City, N.Y.: Anchor, 1984.

Tucker, Lindsay. "Recovering the Conjure Woman: Texts and Contexts in Gloria Naylor's *Mama Day.*" *African American Review* 28.2 (1994): 173–87.

Turner, Victor. *The Ritual Process: Structure and Anti-Structure.* 1969. New York: Aldine de Gruyter, 1995.

Van Dyke, Annette. "From Big Green Fly to the Stone Serpent: Following the Dark Vision in Silko's *Almanac of the Dead.*" *Studies in American Indian Literature* 10.3 (1986): 34–46.

Vaughan, Megan. *Curing Their Ills: Colonial Power and African Illness.* Cambridge: Polity Press, 1991.

Viramontes, Helena. *The Moths and Other Stories.* 1988. Houston: Arte Publico Press, 1997.

———. *Under the Feet of Jesus.* New York: Penguin/Dutton, 1995.

Wagner-Martin, Linda. "Quilting in Gloria Naylor's *Mama Day.*" *Notes on Contemporary Literature* 18.5 (1988): 6–7.

Waitzkin, Howard. *The Politics of Medical Encounters: How Patients and Doctors Deal with Social Problems.* New Haven: Yale University Press, 1991.

Wald, Alan. "The Culture of 'Internal Colonialism': A Marxist Perspective." *MELUS* 8.3 (1981): 18–27.

Walker, Alice. *The Color Purple.* New York: Harcourt Brace Jovanovich, 1982.

———. *Meridian.* San Diego: Harcourt Brace Jovanovich, 1976.

———. *Possessing the Secret of Joy.* New York: Harcourt Brace Jovanovich, 1992.

———. "Strong Horse Tea." In *Love and Trouble,* 88–92. New York: Harcourt, 1973.

———. *The Temple of My Familiar.* New York: Simon and Schuster, 1989.

Warren, Virginia L. "Feminist Directions in Medical Ethics." In *Feminist Perspectives in Medical Ethics,* edited by Helen Bequaert Holmes and Laura M. Purdy, 32–45. Bloomington: Indiana University Press, 1992.

Warshaw, Carole. "Domestic Violence: Challenges to Medical Practice." In *Reframing Women's Health: Multidisciplinary Research and Practice,* edited by Alice J. Dan, 201–18. Thousand Oaks, Calif.: Sage, 1994.

———. "Limitations of the Medical Model in the Care of Battered Women." *Gender and Society* 3.4 (December 1989): 506–17.

White, Evelyn C., ed. *The Black Women's Health Book: Speaking for Ourselves.* Seattle: Seal Press, 1990.

Wilentz, Gay. *Binding Cultures: Black Women Writers in Africa and the Diaspora.* Bloomington: Indiana University Press, 1992.

———. *Healing Narratives: Women Writers Curing Cultural Dis-ease.* New Brunswick, N.J.: Rutgers University Press, 2000.

Williams, D. R., and R. Williams-Morris. "Racism and Mental Health: The African American Experience." *Ethnicity and Health* 5.3–4 (August–November 2000): 243–68.

Winsbro, Bonnie. *Supernatural Forces: Belief, Difference, and Power in Contemporary Works by Ethnic Women.* Amherst: University of Massachusetts Press, 1993.

Wong, Hertha D. "Adoptive Mothers and Throw-Away Children in the Novels of Louise Erdrich." In *Narrating Mothers: Theorizing Maternal Subjectivities,* edited by Brenda O. Daly and Maureen T. Reddy, 174–92. Knoxville: University of Tennessee Press, 1991.

World Health Organization. "Constitution." In *Basic Documents.* 36th ed. Geneva: World Health Organization, 1986.

——. Department of Injuries and Violence Prevention. http://www5.who
    .int/violence—injury—prevention/main.cfm?s=0009.
Yetman, Norman R., ed. *Majority and Minority: The Dynamics of Race and
    Ethnicity in American Life.* 4th ed. Boston: Allyn and Bacon, 1991.
Zaki, Hoda. "Future Tense." *Women's Review of Books* 11.10–11 (July
    1994): 37–38.

Index

261

Permissions

Studies in Social Medicine

Nancy M. P. King, Gail E. Henderson, and Jane Stein, eds., *Beyond Regulations: Ethics in Human Subjects Research* (1999).

Laurie Zoloth, *Health Care and the Ethics of Encounter: A Jewish Discussion of Social Justice* (1999).

Susan M. Reverby, ed. *Tuskegee's Truths: Rethinking the Tuskegee Syphilis Study* (2000).

Beatrix Hoffman, *Wages of Sickness: The Politics of Health Insurance in Progressive America* (2000).

Margarete Sandelowski, *Devices and Desires: Gender, Technology, and American Nursing* (2000).

Keith Wailoo, *Dying in the City of the Blues: Sickle Cell Anemia and the Politics of Race and Health* (2001).

Judith Andre, *Bioethics as Practice* (2002).

Chris Feudtner, *Bittersweet: Diabetes, Insulin, and the Transformation of Illness* (2003).

Ann Folwell Stanford, *Bodies in a Broken World: Women Novelists of Color and the Politics of Medicine* (2003).